Organization Design for Primary Health Care

Noel M. Tichy
foreword by
Amitai Etzioni

The Praeger Special Studies program, through a selective worldwide distribution network, makes available to the academic, government, and business communities significant and timely research in U.S. and international economic, social, and political issues.

Organization Design for Primary Health Care

The Case of the Dr. Martin Luther King, Jr. Health Center

PRAEGER SPECIAL STUDIES IN U.S. ECONOMIC, SOCIAL, AND POLITICAL ISSUES

Praeger Publishers   New York   London

Library of Congress Cataloging in Publication Data

Tichy, Noel M
    Organization design for primary health care.

    (Praeger special studies in U.S. economic, social,
and political issues)
    Bibliography: p.
    Includes index.
    1. Martin Luther King, Jr. Health Center.
2. Community health services—Administration.   I. Title.
RA982.N5M577   362.1'2'09747275   75-44941

PRAEGER SPECIAL STUDIES
200 Park Avenue, New York, N.Y., 10017, U.S.A.

Published in the United States of America in 1977
by Praeger Publishers,
A Division of Holt, Rinehart and Winston, CBS, Inc.

789   038   987654321

To
Monique and Michelle

FOREWORD
Amitai Etzioni

There is a story within Professor Tichy's report on one minority health center and beyond his systematic organizational dissections: a story of participatory effort. The New York City crisis, which sets the background for the current condition of the health center under study, may come and go. Even the national "crisis," the result of runaway inflation of health costs, may one day be reined in. However, interest in efforts and ways to make the governance of health care an area in which lay persons—citizens—can participate, will never go away; it will continue to intrigue experts—and citizens—wherever they are. True, the limelight may be turned elsewhere for a while, making other topics more fashionable. And citizens, preoccupied with the energy shortage, inflation in other areas, or crime, may not talk much or may do little about their role in the management of health care. But the issue is there and will not go away.

Physicians and other health care professionals are viewed as having knowledge superior to that of lay persons and citizens in matters of health. Their authority is not the arbitrary one of power, based on guns, economic accumulation or bureaucratic rank; it is substantive and intrinsic: the authority of knowledge. What room can there be for participation by the untrained? one is often asked.

Health is, at the same time, a matter of value judgments. Should we be more concerned with extension of life than the quality of life we extend? What is the proper balance between preventive and acute care? Is it essential to have a physician of one's own subculture? If funds are short, is it better to have three para-professionals than one doctor? Will lay persons trust their counsel?

These and myriad other questions are largely or wholly value judgments. Once the health implications of the choices involved are clarified, we all can and ought to participate in making these decisions.

The principle is easy; the social mechanisms are hard to come by. Professor Tichy's study does not provide the full answer as to how to allow professionals, semiprofessionals, and citizens—especially those of limited education and under economic pressure—to work together effectively. But his work provides insight into the problem of a minority health center, initiated in an era in which participation was popular, and rich with lessons for an era in which it again will be recognized for what it is: a universal issue.

This book is about the ten-year development of an innovative neighborhood health center in the South Bronx, New York. The managerial and organizational experiences of this center have provided important insights and lessons for primary health care management. To underscore the need for better management and organization design in the primary health care area is to risk being trite. However, the reality is that of the three accepted categories of health care—primary, secondary, and tertiary*—primary care is considered to be the least organized of all medical care (Kissick and Miller, 1976). This is in spite of the fact that the vast majority of health care as measured by the number of people receiving such care is primary care. Out of every 1,000 people on a yearly basis, an average of 720 people receive primary care, 100 people receive secondary care, and 10 receive tertiary care (White, 1973).

Managerially and organizationally, health systems are rarely able to deal with such issues as the optimal mix of scientific knowledge, technology, capital, and personnel for providing service to a definable population market. As Kerr White (1973) points out, these issues are managed quite effectively in the mass production of goods and in delivering such services as transportation and communication. One reason for this disparity is that medical care is a more complex service than most. However, complexity is only one reason why health systems are managerially underdeveloped. Until recently, management expertise was simply kept out of the medical industry. There have been some notable exceptions, including the one discussed in this book.

In the 1960s, the Office of Economic Opportunity (OEO) programs that were geared to help fight the War on Poverty produced many projects that now are frequently maligned as failures and forgotten. But OEO did produce some outstanding successes, including several breakthroughs in the health field that have taught us important and generalizable lessons in the realms of management and organizational

---

*Primary care is treatment based in a physician's office, clinic, ambulatory facility, or health center close to where people live and work. Secondary care is somewhat more specialized consultant care based in fairly large community or district hospitals. Tertiary care is highly specialized, technologically based intensive care, centralized in large medical centers and frequently located in universities (White, 1973).

design. Specifically, the Neighborhood Health Center program generated some extremely innovative primary health care organizations.

Among these neighborhood programs, the Dr. Martin Luther King, Jr. Health Center (henceforth MLK) is a unique case. At MLK, neighborhood workers actually assume managerial responsibilities and are presently directing the center. Although most centers emphasize the hiring and training of indigenous staff for paraprofessional jobs, on the whole there is very little effort to move them into administrative and managerial positions. Yet MLK was able to implement successfully a community management system. This is one of the few cases in which effective community participation was realized in a neighborhood health care center without adversely affecting the delivery of health care. MLK health care is not only patient centered but is also considered by health professionals to be of high technical quality (Morehead, Donaldson, and Servall, 1970).

MLK has been selected as the focus of this book because of the innovations and successes it achieved in several areas of health delivery: MLK is where the collaborative primary health care team has been most extensively and effectively developed as a delivery mechanism for primary health care; MLK developed a unique organizational structure for delivering team-oriented health care; and MLK has evolved from a doctor-controlled organization to one controlled by a community management system.

MLK provided me with my first and most in-depth experience in health care management and organization design. The experience of studying and working with MLK as a researcher and consultant has been accompanied by a deepening and more carefully thought out appreciation for issues of health care management. In developing my current views and feelings toward MLK, I have passed through several phases and have vacillated from singing uncritical praise of MLK to being severely critical of MLK.

As Robert Hollister and co-authors (1974) pointed out, there are two groups of detractors who argue that organizations such as MLK and other OEO neighborhood health centers do not measure up. The first group has been waiting in the wings to pounce on the demonstration projects from their inception. This group includes those with vested interests in the status quo: medical societies, medical school faculties, and bureaucrats. "These criticisms are basically dishonest in that they rue shortcomings for which they are partly responsible and decry failures to reach objectives to which they never before demonstrated allegiance" (Hollister, 1974). The second group of critics is those who supported many of the goals of the center and were often employees. This group is disappointed that its greatest expectation and hopes for the health centers were never met. I was a secret member of this second group for a number of years.

My first introduction to MLK was while teaching a course on organizational change with Richard Beckhard at Columbia University, who used a case study for the students titled "MLK Reorganization." I found the organizational and management issues fascinating, and Beckhard convinced me that health organizations such as MLK were the wave of the future and posed very special and challenging problems for those of us interested in management and organizational behavior.

I, needless to say, became intrigued enough to get involved. Once involved with MLK and a number of other health organizations I began to move through several phases of professional development regarding my perspective. Phase I was one of extreme excitement over the unique characteristics of MLK and its accomplishments in its short history, especially its use of teams and the development of a matrix type of organization. Its goals of providing comprehensive family-oriented care made a great deal of conceptual sense and were congruent with my values.

However, after working with many of the house staff (residents in social medicine) in workshops to provide them with behavioral science skills for team practice, and after conducting a systemwide organizational survey, I gradually became a member of Hollister's second group of detractors. This was phase II of my relationship with MLK. I felt disappointed that MLK was not living up to the expectations and hopes that I had for it. Why wasn't it able to resolve all of its managerial and organizational problems? My standards were very high because, in phase I of my relationship with MLK, my expectations were set unrealistically high. I had felt this was to be *the* model of primary care both at a service delivery level and in terms of its management and organizational design. The reality was, I was discovering, that MLK was "human," it had flaws.

I am now in a new phase in my view of MLK. I have not lost my excitement and sense of idealism regarding the organization. But I have accepted its "humanness" and am now ready to take a more constructively critical stance.

Before continuing, however, I would like to share my biases. I strongly support the goals of MLK: focus on the needs of the poor; a one-door facility, readily accessible in terms of time and place, in which virtually all ambulatory health services are made available; intensive participation by and involvement of the population to be served, both in policy making and as employees; full intetration of and with existing sources of services and funds; assurance of personalized, high-quality care and professional staff of the highest caliber; close coordination with other community resources; and sponsorship by a wide variety of public and private auspices (Schorr and English, 1968, p. 46).

I believe that organizations such as MLK provide one of the most effective vehicles for moving in the direction of accomplishing these goals. However, organizations such as MLK have reached the end of their first decade of existence. The major organizational issues are no longer innovation and new programs, but survival, primarily in terms of financial viability. This is an extremely difficult and trying period for such organizations because they were not brought up to face this kind of world reality. MLK grew up in a protected and affluent environment. Dr. Harold Wise, founder of MLK, always told people, "Don't worry about money, If we want to do it we can get money," and that was the reality—then.

However, as the initial constituencies that had provided support receded, OEO and then HEW (Department of Health, Education, and Welfare) altered their tune and began pressing increasingly for more and more financial self-sufficiency. The process has been gradual, yet the pressure for becoming financially viable is steadily intensifying and, in MLK's case, made worse by New York's financial problems. Already MLK has had to lay off workers and will undoubtedly have to lay off more.

So we have the outstandingly successful neighborhood health center facing issues of survival. There is little chance that MLK will cease operating in the foreseeable future, but there are signs of pressures that can slowly erode the current viability and effectiveness of MLK and eventually transform it into an unrecognizable form.

There are other signs, too, however, that provide a more optimistic view of the future. This book sets out to analyze historically MLK's development and to comment managerially and organizationally on lessons relevant for other health care organizations. For me, personally, it has provided an opportunity to learn and develop to a point where I am now ready to head off to Hazard, Kentucky, to study and help develop a rural comprehensive primary health care system, the Hazard Family Health Services of the Appalachian Regional Hospitals, funded by a grant from the Robert Wood Johnson Foundation. A year from now I will begin work on the rural counterpart to the MLK case.

ACKNOWLEDGMENTS

Now that this book is completed, I can reflect on how the task was accomplished. In so doing it becomes clear that I owe a debt of gratitude to several people and to the Grace Foundation.

I am especially grateful to the Grace Foundation for providing me with a one-year Grace Fellowship at the Graduate School of Business, Columbia University, which enabled me to carry out the major work on the book.

I am indebted to Richard Beckhard, of MIT's Sloan School of Management, who convinced me that managerial and organizational issues in the health field were stimulating and challenging. It was through his contact with the Dr. Martin Luther King Health Center that I became involved in this project in the first place. He has continued to provide support and encouragement all along the way.

I am also indebted to several of my colleagues at Columbia University who provided both encouragement and useful comments on various drafts of the manuscript. Eli Ginzberg provided both intellectual and financial research support for my initial work with the Dr. Martin Luther King Health Center, and continues to push me to look at the broader policy issues in the health field. Michael Tushman provided useful feedback on an early version of the manuscript. Amitai Etzioni continues to be a source of intellectual and moral support. Finally, I owe a special debt of gratitude to my friend and colleague, Charles Kadushin, who is somehow always magically able to take my rough and often muddled early drafts and help me sort out the important issues from the trivial.

Irwin Rubin was also critical in helping me. His frank and honest critique of an early version resulted in stimulating me to rewrite the book totally.

I owe a debt of gratitude to many if not most of the people at the Dr. Martin Luther King, Jr. Health Center who over the last few years have been extremely open, supportive, and cooperative. I have made many friends there and am especially thankful of the support of the management group, Kathleen Estrada, William Lloyd, Elinor Minor, Gloria Perry, Deloris Smith, and Sonia Valdez.

Last, but most important, I must thank Monique Tichy, without whose comments, support, patience, and love I never would have completed this book.

CONTENTS

LIST OF TABLES AND FIGURES

Organization Design for Primary Health Care

1

FROM INNOVATION
TO SURVIVAL:
MANAGERIAL AND
ORGANIZATIONAL LESSONS

The Dr. Martin Luther King, Jr. Health Center (MLK) is a neighborhood health center originally sponsored by the Office of Economic Opportunity (OEO) under Section 314(c) of the Partnership in Health Act, which has been transferred for continuing support to the Department of Health, Education, and Welfare (HEW). As such, it was established as one of over 140 such centers across the country as a demonstration project (Hollister, Kramer, and Bellin, 1974). The general charge was for the centers to develop a community-based health program to provide a spectrum of medical and health-related services to a defined population. There was to be maximum feasible participation of local residents, including recruiting and training as health workers to provide the center's services.

The Martin Luther King, Jr. Health Center has a very impressive list of accomplishments and has certainly provided an innovative setting for new developments in primary care. Before some of these accomplishments are presented, one of the basic contradictions and dilemmas facing MLK (and one of the themes of this book) will be identified.

MLK is no longer primarily a demonstration project. It is an institution providing service to a poverty community. No longer is federal money made available to stimulate innovations. This money now arrives tagged with the message to get the ship in order so that it will become more financially self-sufficient. How does an organization that had a great infusion of money and of creative talent whose initial purpose for being seems to have been to make some people's dreams come true and that accomplished many of these dreams make the transition to a financially self-sufficient, viable institution in an environment such as that of New

1

York? New York is a city whose municipal hospitals are being forced to close and whose giant private medical centers, such as Montefiore Hospital and Medical Center under whose auspices MLK functions, are facing considerable financial uncertainties.

One reason why institutions such as MLK find themselves in such severe difficulties is that the economic world has changed and with it some of the basic ground rules. The basic rules in the mid-1960s were geared to provide innovative services in areas of need; in the mid-1970s, the rules are being geared to promote financial viability.

In part, this change in rules represents a societal "dirty trick" on some very novel service organizations started by OEO. The War on Poverty created expectations that social and health problems could and would be ameliorated via a massive infusion of federal resources into areas of high need. These expectations have had to be postponed or even quashed.

Let us examine the guiding assumptions of the early OEO neighborhood health centers: geograhic area of high need; need for comprehensive services; innovative and experimental; significant involvement of community members and patients who are to receive health care.

There was no explicit demand to operate these programs like a business; in other words, there was no requirement to measure market share, return on investment, cost effectiveness, and so on. Figure 1.1

FIGURE 1.1

Driving Forces Guiding Neighborhood Health Center OEO (HEW) Funding Strategy

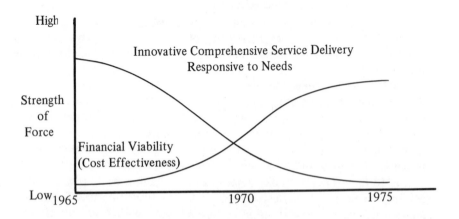

Source: Compiled by the author.

shows the dominant force behind OEO funding in 1965 to be innovative service delivery, with financial viability playing an almost nonexistent role. As a result, those who were granted funds in the early OEO days were by and large liberal, social-change-minded innovators looking to fight the War on Poverty. The good ones, such as Dr. Harold Wise, founder of MLK, were social entrepreneurs who had visions of a better way of delivering health care. Most of these social-change entrepreneurs had no desire to deal with financing such programs other than through grants. Society, via OEO, allowed these great expectations for social change to be raised by encouraging the Harold Wises of the 1960s to be creative and expansive without regard to long-term financial self-sufficiency. In spite of the lack of direct concern with cost effectiveness on the part of some founders, such as Dr. Wise, studies have demonstrated that "on an average unit-cost basis, the neighborhood health center is considered competitive on unit costs to other alternative institutional providers" (Sparer and Anderson, 1972).

The dirty trick was to change the ground rules in midstream without adequate preparation. From innovation and the implementation of needed services, the criteria shifted to financial self-sufficiency and cost effectiveness with little regard for the original service-oriented concept. The shift in the emphasis from innovativeness to financial viability, however, did come gradually, even though the impact was felt quite dramatically in the early 1970s. There always were individuals in the background pushing for a balance between the two differing forces. It was not, however, until the early 1970s that the two forces balanced each other. By the mid-1970s, the financial viability force far outweighed the innovative force. The ground rules became consolidation for efficiency, cost effectiveness, financial accountability to funding sources, and eventual self-sufficiency.

With hindsight, it is clear that these two forces are both legitimate and, although somewhat conflicting, not mutually exclusive. The dirty trick was that government did not acknowledge this from the outset and therefore did not initiate a systematic approach needed to balance the idealistic-innovative approach in the project's early days against realistic cost-effectiveness requirements. If this had occurred, it might have been possible to have avoided an extreme, and painful, swing from one orientation to the other.

MLK has been greatly affected during its development by these two forces. This will be demonstrated in this book and is reflected in the following quote from Deloris Smith, current director of the center, who stated in 1973 that:

> My dream is to create a consumer education program that would allow patients to participate in their own health care process. The approach would include the involvement of patients and health providers as co-

partners in the health care delivery process. The patient would be primarily responsible for his own health status. The health provider's role would become a supportive one, but the patient would assume most of the responsibility.

Ms. Smith also predicted that:

In the next year we will be formalizing many demonstration projects we have developed over the past seven years. . . . These projects will be offered to other health centers and ambulatory facilities. I view MLK becoming a technical and consultation service for other ambulatory-care facilities. With the Health Maintenance Organization plan fully developed and the almost certain likelihood of national health insurance, the Center's services will be secured (Smith, 1973).

Three short years later, Deloris Smith still has similar dreams (as shown in Chapter 9). However, nothing seems certain. In the three intervening years, there have been layoffs, a declining population base, and severe financial constraints because of federal, state, and city pressures. In fact, MLK currently is stalled on the way to fulfilling its dreams.

MLK's experience is not uncommon. Generally, when organizations are created, there is an initial phase of entrepreneurial activity. Usually, this is spearheaded by a charismatic leader or leadership group. However, there comes a point in the development of most organizations where they face a developmental crisis, that of moving beyond the entrepreneurial phase. Larry Greiner (1972) labels this the "creativity phase." In the case of MLK, this crisis may also be associated with a changed environment.

A deeper appreciation and understanding of the dynamics of this process and the organizational and managerial implications are called for in the health field, for it is clear that the scenario will be replayed many times as both government and private foundations continue to stimulate the development of new health organizations. Recent examples are HEW's Rural Initiative Project, the pending federally sponsored Health Maintenance Organizations, the Robert Wood Johnson Foundation's Rural Practice Project, and the HEW-sponsored Urban Initiative Project.

In analyzing the MLK case, it is hoped that new insights can be gleaned that will contribute to policies and managerial practices whose function would be to make it easier for new primary health organizations to shift from the creativity phase to viability in the real world.

Viability in the real world will be defined as functioning as a "healthy" organization, one that does more than merely survive. This is because an organization can survive for years as it slowly dies. This slow deterioration is referred to as the entropic process. "The entropic process is a universal law of nature in which all forms of organization move toward disorganization and death" (Katz and Kahn, 1966, p. 21). A "healthy" organization is characterized as one that, in Daniel Katz and Robert Kahn's terms, can acquire negative entropy, which entails importing more energy from its environment than it expends and storing it (1966, p. 21). Negative entropy is one facet of the key determinant of organizational health, namely, the existence of self-renewal capability, which also consists of processes that help the organization develop better ways of conserving and utilizing energy (people, capital, and technology). The MLK case study traces the development of MLK with an eye on the forces that lead to self-renewal capability.

BACKGROUND OF MLK

The founder of the project was Dr. Harold Wise, originally on the staff of the Montefiore Department of Social Medicine. This department was known as a focal point for socially concerned physicians. The MLK project was in fact a culmination of earlier efforts within the department to reform the delivery of health care in the South Bronx (Silver, 1963).

MLK serves one of the most blighted urban areas in the United States. The problems of deteriorating housing, widespread unemployment, lack of educational opportunity, crime, and drugs have contributed to a complex of socially related health problems that defy a conventional medical solution.

The center was funded in 1966 as a result of an OEO grant administered by Montefiore Hospital and Medical Center, a voluntary hospital located several miles from MLK in a middle-income section of the Bronx. Montefiore enjoys considerable prestige, not only as a highly regarded teaching hospital but also as a developer of innovative health delivery systems.

MLK provides comprehensive primary health services to 39,000 residents of one section of the South Bronx in which there are 75,000 residents. The neighborhood has a racial makeup of 62 percent black, 36 percent Puerto Rican, and 2 percent other (see Appendix B for an historical fact sheet and budget data on MLK).

The services offered by MLK include four levels of care as defined by Gerald Sparer and Andre Anderson (1972):

1. First level: primary clinical medical care, consisting of four basic units: medical, x-ray, laboratory, and pharmacy.

2. Second level: primary medical care, including the first level of care, plus home health and mental health.
3. Third level: primary comprehensive medical care, including the second level, combined with supporting health services (social and community services, training, transportation, community organization, and research and evaluation).
4. Fourth level: primary comprehensive health care, including the third level, plus dental care. (See Appendix A for a more detailed breakdown of services as well as a patient and financial breakdown for MLK from 1966 to 1976.)

The main building is a five-story renovated warehouse located between a school and a supermarket; it faces a massive housing project that is a landmark in the area. The center has a storefront look, providing for easy patient access. The ambience is cheerful and nonhospital, in marked contrast to the style of charity medicine prevailing in the wards of hospitals in urban settings. Visitors often comment on the apparent rapport between staff and patients. The overall impression is that the center is integrated into the life of the community. (See Appendix B for a floor plan.)

Government funding, now in the form of an HEW grant, covers about half of the approximately $8 million budget of the center. Reimbursements for medical services through various programs, such as Medicaid, Medicare, Blue Shield, and GHI, provide additional support (see Appendix B for the financial history of MLK in some detail).

Since its founding, the center has relied on the resources of Montefiore Hospital. Dr. Wise was a member of the hospital's innovative Department of Social Medicine. Dr. Martin Cherkasky, director of Montefiore Hospital and Medical Center, has been in the forefront of reform within the medical establishment. He provided the center with a base of support during its development. As the transition from hospital to community management took place, there was a transfer of knowledge, skills, legitimacy, and power from a small group of Montefiore physicians to a carefully selected and trained group of community health workers. At present (early 1977), the administrative responsibilities still vested in the Montefiore management are minimal. But the hospital is still the fiscal agent for the supporting grant.

ORGANIZATIONAL STRUCTURE OF THE CENTER

MLK is a predominantly "normative" type of organization (Etzioni, 1961), meaning that the organization elicits involvement and exercises control through the use of such factors as membership, status, and intrinsic rewards. Amitai Etzioni points out that in such organizations the members tend to value intrinsically the mission of the organization and their jobs within it. Performance and compliance occur because there is a moral and value commitment on the part of members. The ten-year development of MLK shows how a predominantly normative organization evolves to become a complex mixture of normative and utilitarian. "Utilitarian" organizations are those in which people perform and comply largely because of payment, and the exercise of authority is rational-legal in nature, not value oriented. Many of the internal developments and dilemmas at MLK can be explained in terms of the shifts from an organization in which members started out with a predominantly moral involvement to one where many members developed a calculative involvement. This development is followed as a theme in the remainder of this book.

The MLK system is more egalitarian than the traditional physician-controlled system; power is more equally distributed and there has been considerably more career mobility for nonprofessionals from the community. Prescriptive barriers to career progress, such as ethnicity, social class, or sex, have been removed. The center has provided a greater variety of career opportunities than traditional health institutions and has given many community workers a second chance in their professional lives. It has developed innovative training programs and flexible career ladders that have sidestepped the traditional health credentialing system, which generally restricts indigenous workers to very limited tracks. The present top and middle managers were initially employed in paraprofessional positions at the center. Most are minority women over 30 who had no previous technical training or education beyond high school when they started at MLK.

Although MLK is more egalitarian than the traditional system, it is, nonetheless, stratified and hierarchical. There is no worker-management structure in which formal mechanisms such as elected managers and worker board representation exist, which was initially one of Dr. Wise's dreams. The present top and middle managers exercise a bureaucratic type of authority and have progressed further in their education and training than most of the other workers. As indicated above, MLK's compliance system has evolved from predominantly normative to mixed normative and utilitarian (use of rational-legal authority, use of economic rewards—Etzioni, 1961).

THE HEALTH TEAMS

MLK is organized around collaborative health teams. While health teams are increasingly used to deliver care in the United States, their internal structure often has tended to replicate that of the hospital hierarchy. The MLK teams, on the other hand, have attracted national attention as a new, more collaborative model of delivery, in a departure from the physician-dominated system. Power is redistributed as family health workers carry out some of the traditional roles of nurses, and nurse practitioners have assumed many of the physicans' responsibilities.

The MLK collaborative teams were developed before the community management system, and served as a model for professional-paraprofessional cooperation in the delivery of health care. Several of the top and middle managers were family health care workers on the teams, and many of the critical mentor relationships between physicians and current managers developed within the team framework.

MANAGEMENT

In the ten years since its founding, MLK has evolved from a traditional professional type of organization dominated by physicians (Etzioni, 1969; Friedson, 1970) to a distinctly new and more bureaucratic type of organization directed by community managers. Figure 1.2 depicts the organizational structure of the traditional type of health center, which is based on that of the hospital. Figure 1.3 shows the current organization of MLK.

There are two levels of management. The top group of six has four individuals from the community who worked their way up through the MLK organization. The project director and the administrator were both in the first group of family health workers. The director of health services was one of the first employees in the MLK Medical Records Department. The former director of training, now head of the Bathgate Satellite Clinic, is a public health nurse with many years of community-oriented experience in the area. The assistant director of health services is an internist who has been with MLK since its beginning, and was formerly project director. He is the only physician in the top group. He is also the only male.

Middle management is composed of persons who have moved up from lower level positions at the center. Seven unit managers make up the largest middle-management group. Team members are supervised by unit managers in administrative matters. Almost all of the top and middle managers are black or Puerto Rican women.

There are also professional supervisors for nursing, internal medicine, pediatrics, and family health workers. These supervisors report to the director of health services. They do not have formal administrative authority. Their influence is solely in the professional clinical area.

FIGURE 1.2

Traditional Organizational Chart

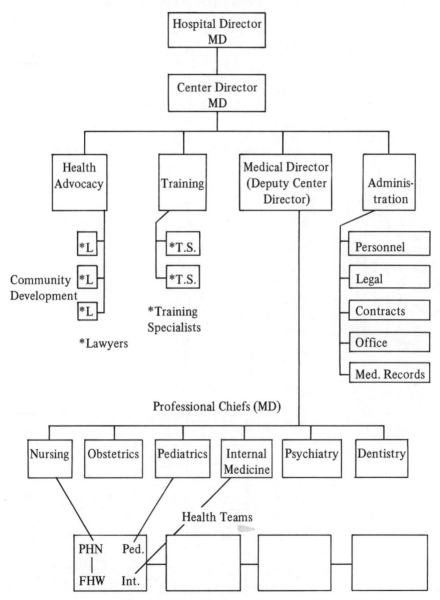

Source: Harold Wise, Richard Beckhard, Irwin Rubin, and Aileen L. Kyte, *Making Health Teams Work* (Cambridge, Mass.: Ballinger, 1974).

FIGURE 1.3
Martin Luther King, Jr. Health Center
Organizational Chart

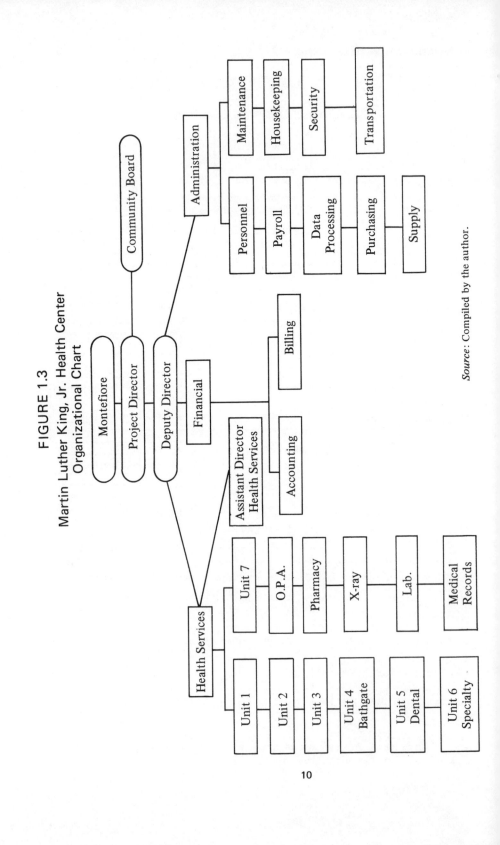

Source: Compiled by the author.

ACCOMPLISHMENTS ALONG THE WAY

MLK became a leader in the primary care field due to the following accomplishments:

The development of the family-oriented comprehensive primary health care team (Wise et al., 1974).

The development and utilization of community (family) health workers.

The development and utilization of primary care nurse practitioners.

The development of an organization structure to support team delivery of care (use of a matrix design introduced by Richard Beckhard [1972] of MIT's Sloan School of Management).

A large-scale job-training program for community members for health-related jobs both within and outside MLK.

The development of a Patient Bill of Rights.

An internal structure managed by community members. In this, top and middle managers are predominantly indigenous and promoted from lower positions in MLK (see Chapter 4).

Perhaps most important of all is the fact that the quality of care at MLK is considered superior. In a study in which MLK scored above average in quality for neighborhood health centers, "The conclusion reached from review of this data [a comparison of audits in 35 neighborhood health centers versus 52 other providers] is that at the present time . . . the neighborhood health center program performance is equal to and in some instances superior to that of other established providers of health care" (Morehead, Donaldson, and Sexavalli, 1971).

EFFECT ON OTHER INSTITUTIONS

By following the progress of people who took part in the early years of MLK's development, one can trace the ripple effect of MLK on other institutions. To find and train physicians who were willing and able to function in a team setting, Harold Wise started an Internship and Residency Program in Social Medicine at Montefiore Hospital. This program attracted a self-selected group of physicians who wanted the MLK experience as part of their training. The residents in this program spent aproximately half of their clinical time practicing at MLK.

Another serendipitous set of circumstances brought about MLK's impact on MIT's Sloan School of Management. When Harold Wise experienced managerial and organizational problems in 1970, he turned to Margaret Mahoney, then at Carnegie Foundation, for advice. She, in turn, referred him to a colleague, Richard Beckhard of MIT's Sloan

School of Management. This was Beckhard's first experience with health organizations. In addition to having a profound impact on MLK in terms of improving the teams and redesigning the organization, the experience stimulated Beckhard and his colleagues to focus their attention on health care organizations. As a result, MIT's Sloan School of Management is deeply involved in health care management and, in collaboration with the American Association of Medical Colleges, has initiated a management training program for deans of medical centers.

Another outgrowth of MLK is the Institute for Health Team Development funded by the Robert Wood Johnson Foundation. This institute was established in 1974 by Harold Wise, along with Richard Beckhard, David Kindig, and Dr. Jo Boufford (the latter two were residents in the Social Medicine Program). Its role is to provide primary care team education within health science centers. The institute developed primary care curricula and organized faculty teams at four university health science centers across the country. In addition, it established the Valentine Lane Family Practice, which is a primary health care team practicing in Yonkers, New York. Three of the professional staff of Valentine Lane: the pediatrician, Dr. Bihari, the internist, Dr. Leicht, the nurse practitioner, Ms. Uribelarrea, were former MLK employees; the fourth, a social worker, Ms. Ulrich, was not a former MLK employee.

Another institute that has its origins in the MLK experience is the Lehman-Montefiore Health Professions Institute, which is training primary care nurse practitioners, social workers, and medical service administrators at the baccalaureate level.

MLK also has had substantial indirect impact on primary health care in other organizations, through the flow of young physicians who have passed through MLK in training. Included in this group are the past two heads of the National Health Service Core, one of whom moved on to be head of Health Manpower at HEW. He is currently director of Montefiore Hospital and Medical Center.

As an OEO demonstration project, MLK may not have met the highest expectations, but in relation to other OEO neighborhood health centers it has certainly achieved a unique impact in important aspects of primary care.

RECENT DEVELOPMENTS

As the initial constituencies that had provided support for MLK began to recede in importance, OEO and then HEW altered their approach and began pressing for more and more financial self-sufficiency.

The process has been gradual, yet the pressure for optimal financial effectiveness is steadily intensifying, and MLK's overall situation is worsened by New York's fiscal problems. Already, MLK has had to lay off workers and may have to lay off more.

Thus, we have a picture of an outstandingly successful neighborhood health center facing serious problems of survival. There is little chance that MLK will cease operating in the foreseeable future. But certain pressures may slowly erode the current effectiveness of MLK and may eventually turn it into an ineffective organism, dominated by the entire process. These pressures, a major focus of the remaining chapters, include a decreasing patient population base, a slow retreat from the primary care team concept back to physician-dominated care, an increasing cleavage between staff and management, decreasing resources and managerial support for innovations, layoffs, and a decreased sense of idealism and unifying organizational goals and mission.

This book sets out to discuss the organizational behavior and managerial aspects of MLK's development and its current organizational dilemmas. The book will be built around an organizational framework presented in Chapter 2. The remaining chapters focus on different organizational components—how they developed, their current form, as well as an assessment of their strengths and weaknesses and the implications for improved organizational effectiveness.

2

AN ORGANIZATIONAL
FRAMEWORK:
MLK'S ORGANIZATIONAL
DILEMMAS

The usual organization pursues a superficial image of rationality which understates the value of imperfection. Not only can every organization expect imperfection, a self-designing organization should seek it. An optimal degree of imperfection attaches no more certainty to assumptions than their credibility deserves, converts imbalances into motivators, and uses unclear goals to keep an organization as ready for change as its environment is. . . .

A self-designing organization can attain dynamic balances through overlapping, unplanned, and non-rational proliferations of its processes; and these proliferating processes collide, contest, and interact with one another to generate wisdom. (B. Hedberg, P. Nystrom, and W. Starbuck, "Camping on Seesaws: Prescriptions for a Self-Designing Organization," *Administrative Science Quarterly* 21, no. 1 [March 1976], p.63.)

The case analysis of the Dr. Martin Luther King, Jr. Health Center is guided by a simple yet comprehensive framework for diagnosing and understanding complex organizations. The framework and its components reflect contemporary developments in the organizational behavior and managerial fields. A central guiding theme reflected in the framework and developed in each chapter of this book is that the practice of management and the design of organizations consist, to a large extent, of balancing a set of often paradoxical, sometimes rational and sometimes nonrational, processes (Hedberg, Nystrom, and Starbuck, 1976). These processes require constant attention to what will be shown as trade-offs between two evils or between two desired ends.

Organizations and managers are engaged in a dynamic balancing act. The successful manager in a complex organization, such as MLK, needs to thrive on paradoxes. These paradoxes at MLK are reflected in such tradeoffs as balancing the advantages and disadvantages of rationally developing strategic plans versus muddling through; being too flexible versus being too rigid; attending to quality of care versus attending to quantity of care; investment in people versus investment in the system; and encouraging conformity versus encouraging dissension.

Each component of the framework has associated with it several dilemmas or trade-offs that are of particular importance in the analysis of MLK. The framework and these trade-offs are highlighted in the remainder of this chapter.

SOME DIMENSIONS OF ORGANIZATIONAL LIFE: A FRAMEWORK

In the most abstract sense, primary health care organizations are not different from other organizations, large or small, business or service. Indeed we would be most unwise if in our excitement over the challenges of dealing with primary health organizations we lost sight of their commolities with other social organizations. The commonalities create a backdrop against which some unique aspects of primary health care organizations can be compared. For this reason some of the universal dimensions of organizational life are presented.

In considering primary health care organizations, such as MLK, we will place different emphasis on some of the dimensions and their relationships with other dimensions. Figure 2.1 depicts the framework. Each of the dimensions of organizational life is identified. The overall scheme emphasizes the concept of an organization as a dynamic entity in constant interaction with its environment—absorbing inputs and transforming them into outputs to the external environment. MLK takes in patients (inputs) and provides services (transformation process) that alter the health status (outputs) of the patients (with an effect on the environment that eventually leads to feedback for MLK) (Katz and Kahn, 1966).

Environment

Organizations are greatly influenced by the environment within which they operate. The environment provides the opportunities as well as the constraints for the organization. The problem for management is to choose among these constraints and opportunities. The criteria for the choices are developed from management's perception of the organization's purpose: its raison d'etre, its mission. For example there are

FIGURE 2.1

Organizational Model

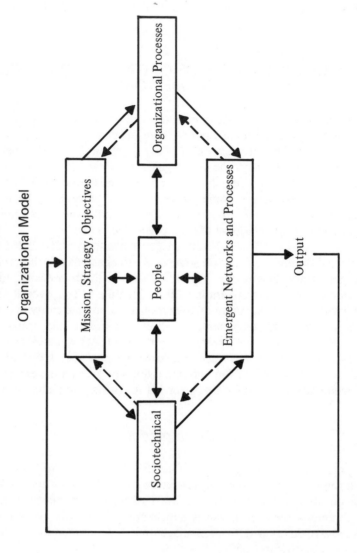

Source: Compiled by the author.

important managerial and organizational differences between a neighbor-hood health center that has a mission of innovation in primary health care and one whose mission is to provide basic health services to the largest possible number of community residents. The two would have different staffing patterns and would offer different health services.

Steven Shortell (1976) identified five dimensions of the environment that have implications for organizational design responses. The environmental categories are presented in Table 2.1 along with a summary of MLK's environment in each category in 1967 and in 1977.

As Table 2.1 indicates, MLK's environment has moved toward greater complexity (more forces to deal with), greater diversity (more different forces to deal with), lower stability stability (changing more rapidly), and higher uncertainty (cannot predict changes as easily), while its dependence on Montefiore Hospital and HEW has remained constant. Therefore, in Shortell's terms there have been shifts in both the content of the environment and in its very nature, resulting in a relatively intense environment.

Some of the environmental factors that contribute to making it intense are the uncertainty over New York State Medicaid rates, New York City's faltering on the brink of bankruptcy, possible changes in HEW funding, the imminent transfer of the HEW grant to a community and consumer board, Montefiore's financial cutbacks, the erosion of the population base in the South Bronx in MLK's catchment area, and the "Medicaid mills" that are providing direct competition for MLK.

Given this type of environment, organization research indicates that the design of the organization most appropriate to effective functioning is relatively organic (Burns and Stalker, 1961; Lawrence and Lorsch, 1967), characterized by the following (Tushman and Nadler, 1976):

Low formalization (Hage and Aiken, 1967): low specification of the tasks in terms of rules, standard operating procedures, policies, and so on
Decentralization: participative decision-making structure, a structure that involves lower level organization members in a high percentage of decisions
Differentiated reward structure: use of multiple diverse arrangements to induce members to carry out work
Nonprogrammed coordination: application of personal and group or team methods to coordinate work
Nonprogrammed control: relatively large use of personal and group methods to obtain feedback and evaluate performance by means of personal meetings and group conferences

As will be discussed in later chapters, MLK's organization design does not totally match these prescriptions, which in part explains some of the organizational difficulties experienced by MLK.

TABLE 2.1

Typology of Environmental Dimensions

	Content of Environment			
	Low Complexity		High Complexity	
Nature of Environment	Low Diversity	High Diversity	Low Diversity	High Diversity
Stability:				
High predictability of occurrence — High predictability of content	1966			
Low predictability of content				
Low predictability of occurrence — High predictability of content				
Low predictability of content				
Instability				
High predictability of occurrence — High predictability of content				
Low predictability of content				
Low predictability of occurrence — High predictability of content				
Low predictability of content				1977

Source: Steven Shortell, "The Role of Environment in a Configurational Theory of Organizations," *Human Relations* 30 (1977): 280.

Mission, Strategy, and Objectives

The administrator in complex organizations must guide the organization through the making of choices among apparently equal priorities in order to develop criteria for an organizational strategy. (Strategy is the process of setting goals and obectives in the context of the organization's mission.) The goals and obectives provide a set of targets and controls necessary in order to achieve the mission.

Every organization has a mission, strategy, and obectives. They may not be clear and people may behave in ways that are inconsistent with them, but they exist nonetheless. The analysis of MLK's strategy is divided into three areas: health service strategy, environment strategy, and administrative strategy. Each area is examined over the ten-year period.

Sociotechnical Arrangements

The component in Figure 2.1 labeled "sociotechnical" refers to the technology by which the organization's work is carried out and to the social structure necessary to operate that technology. The technology of work (in the case of MLK's various medical procedures) limits the way in which an organization becomes structured but does not totally determine the final structure.

Two aspects of technology are considered important in determining structure: How many exceptions are there? That is, to what degree do nonroutine problems arise? For example, most surgical teams have routine technologies with few exceptions, compared to a primary care health team where exceptions abound. And once there is an exception, to what extent can the solution be analyzed? Are ready-made solutions or contingency plans available? These plans exist when certain things go wrong in surgery, but there are often no contingency plans for exceptions in primary care (Perrow, 1965). An example of a nonroutine and unanalyzable situation in primary care is when a family member exhibits an unusual combination of physical and psychosocial symptoms. The search for a solution becomes unique.

As the technology varies in these two areas so does the structure most appropriate to effective functioning. Another factor in determining the appropriate structure is how individuals will respond (some do well in highly formal and prescribed situations while others need more flexibility and discretion).

As Figure 2.1 implies, the particular sociotechnical arrangement flows in part from the mission, strategy, and objectives of the organization. But it is also influenced by the other components of the framework. The central issue related to sociotechnical arrangements is how best to organize work so as to optimize both human and technological effectiveness.

Organizational Processes

In addition to sociotechnical arrangements, the organization needs a series of mechanisms that enable the sociotechnical system to perform its work. These mechanisms are called organizational processes. They include communication processes, control processes, problem-solving and decision-making processes, and conflict management processes.

Communication: The key organizational issues with regard to communication are to develop procedures for minimal distortion, minimal time lag, and sufficient openness to facilitate upward and downward communication.

Control: Organizations require control structures for regulating performance (Etzioni, 1975; Lawler, 1976). Unfortunately, all too often control systems foster dysfunctional organizational behavior and are known for encouraging number game playing (Blau, 1955). The analysis of the MLK case focuses on both the functional and dysfunctional aspects of its control system.

Problem solving and decision making. Organizations such as MLK need to develop multiple methods for solving problems. For example, mechanisms are needed to guide clinical problem solving and decision making, whereas different mechanisms are needed to coordinate allocation of organizational resources and for routine administrative decisions.

Reward systems: Research has shown that there is often a discrepancy between what organizations aspire to reward and what in fact they do reward (Lawler, 1976). The challenge to MLK is to develop a reward system that rewards behavior that enhances organizational objectives while at the same time recognizing and rewarding differences between groups and individuals.

Conflict management: Organizational conflict is an inevitable phenomenon occurring at individual, interpersonal, intergroup, and organizational levels Processes need to be available for diagnosing and managing it in order to avoid dysfunctional consequences and to enhance the potential for obtaining some of its benefits (Deutsch, 1973; Walton, 1969).

People

Most importantly, organizations have people who operate within sociotechnical structures and operate the organizational processes. It is people whose behavior is both determined by and who in turn determine mission, strategy, and objectives; sociotechnical arrangements; organizational processes; and emergent networks and processes.

Emergent Networks and Processes

The preceding discussion of sociotechnical arrangements and organizational processes implies that these arrangements are somehow totally formally prescribed and rationally planned. As has been recognized for years (Sayles, 1958), this is not so. Systems develop extensive informal structures and processes that emerge as a result of human interaction in the organization (Blau, 1955; Blau, 1956). Figure 2.1 focuses on both the formal arrangements and processes and the informal or emergent ones.

These networks of relationships and processes emerge because individuals tend to formulate, reformulate, and interpret the mission; understand, abide by, and/or change the formal sociotechnical arrangements and organizational processes; use, abuse, and alter the technology; and differentially respond to changing environmental conditions. As a result, a new set of unplanned and often unanticipated structures and processes perforce affects the course of decision making, problem solving, leadership, power distribution, and so on (Hornstein and Tichy, 1976; Weick, 1969).

These unplanned structures and processes are needed to get the work done, especially in organizations such as MLK, which are so complex that blueprints or plans can never be developed for all contingencies. Unplanned structures emerge to get the work done, ranging from simple informal case conferences in the hallways between nurse practitioners and physicians to more complex coalitions formed to develop new health services for the total agency. These unplanned processes have potentially double-edged consequences. They may either facilitate or hinder the accomplishment of an organization's mission. Although not the focus of a separate chapter, emergent networks and processes are dealt with throughout the book.

TABLE 2.2

Greiner's Model of Organization Growth as Applied to Health Centers

	Phase 1 Growth Through Creativity	Phase 2 Growth Through Direction	Phase 3 Growth Through Delegation	Phase 4 Growth Through Coordination	Phase 5 Growth Through Collaboration
Management focus	Develop new form of health delivery	Efficiency of operations	Expansion	Consolidation of organizations	Problem solving and innovation
Organization structure	Informal (emergent)	Centralized and functional	Decentralized and geographic	Line staff and service groups	Matrix of teams
Top management style	Individualistic and entrepreneurial	Directive	Delegative	Watchdog	Participative
Control system	Feedback from community and patients	Standards and cost centers (teams and units)	Reports and profit centers	Plans and investment centers	Mutual goal setting
Management reward emphasis	Salary and feeling of "owning" new innovations	Salary and merit increases	Individual bonus	Profit sharing (cost-saving sharing)	Team bonus
		Crisis of Leadership ↑	Crisis of Autonomy ↑	Crisis of Control ↑	Crisis of Red Tape ↑

Source: Adapted from Larry Greiner, "Evolution and Revolution as Organizations Grow," *Harvard Business Review* (July-August 1972).

Organizational Outputs

The framework also focuses on organizational outputs. These include outputs directly related to organizational objectives, such as the quality and quantity of patient care, as well as outputs relative to organizational members, their behavior, and satisfaction. The feedback loop (see Figure 2.1) provides the information necessary for the organization to adapt to the consequences of its output.

The Time Factor

The framework just presented provides a way of examining important components of an organization. But it lacks another important factor, that of time. Organizations develop over time and pass through a number of developmental stages. Although there is a paucity of research on the exact nature of the phases of organizational development and growth, the concept has been evident in the writings of Max Weber on bureaucracy (1946) and is dealt with by Alfred Chandler (1962), William Newman and J.P. Logan (1955), and Larry Greiner (1972).

Greiner's (1972) formulation is employed in analyzing the case of MLK. Table 2.2 summarizes Greiner's model, modified for application to neighborhood health centers. The framework presented in Figure 2.1 provides the basic organization of this book. Examination of the components will center on the identification of critical dilemmas and trade-offs that were both significant in the development of MLK and that are of importance in the management and organization design of other primary care health systems. The next section of this chapter briefly presents the dilemmas associated with each of the framework's components.

DILEMMAS: TRADE-OFFS IN DESIGNING AND MANAGING PRIMARY CARE

Obviously, many of the dilemmas that MLK faces will not have direct relevance and application to other primary care systems. However, many will. The final chapter of this book will address the issue of generalization from the MLK case to other organizations.

The dilemmas dealt with in this book are portrayed figuratively as scales that require balancing. This is to create the image of management and organization design as a dynamic process requiring careful weighing of many, often conflicting, issues (Weick, 1969). Management is faced with the task of monitoring the scales, rebalancing them when a disturbance comes along to knock them off balance, and planning for ways to keep them balanced in the future. Table 2.3 presents a list of the major dilemmas that MLK has faced in each component of the framework and that will be treated as scales throughout this book. These dilemmas are briefly discussed below.

Environment

Most of the scales located outside the organization relate to how MLK balances conflicting environmental demands for community participation and control. The other area of the environment of relevance is that of health financing. Balancing the scales in this area involves such tradeoffs as local Bronx political agendas versus city, state, and federal political agendas being met; Montefiore as paternalistic protector versus MLK's independence; middle-class norms and behavior on the board versus poverty-class norms and behavior on the board; external community control of the center versus community control via a system of management filled with community people; and reimbursement realities versus what the patients really need in the way of services.

Mission, Strategy, and Objectives

In 1973 the goals of MLK were formally set down in its annual report: to provide health care that is family-centered and comprehensive; to provide health center staff with skills to improve work performance and upgrading for work in the health field; to involve community residents in health education projects to improve the community health status; and to build a system of care so effective that it can be copied elsewhere.

A study carried out by the author in January 1974 in which 60 percent (234) of the staff responded indicated that organization members' views of the goals varied (see Table 2.4). For example, management's priorities were different from the average organization member's priority ratings. The differences become even more striking when the responses of people from Unit 1 are compared to management's ratings. MLK, therefore, is an organization with a set of formal written goals that are not consistent with the organization members' perceptions of the goals. Although the lack of consensus about goals is not unusual in a complex organization (March and Simon, 1958; Perrow, 1970), it does pose some organizational dilemmas.

Lack of goal consensus makes it more difficult for goals to serve the functions identified by Etzioni (1975), which are to focus energy and act

TABLE 2.3

Organizational Dilemmas

Component	Dilemmas: Trade-offs Requiring Balancing
External interface	Local politics versus state and federal
	Montefiore as paternalistic provider versus independence
	External community control versus internal management
	Elite cooptation versus radical egalitarianism
	Middle-class norms and behavior versus poverty-class norms and behavior
Mission, strategy, objectives	
Mission	High faith versus minimal faith
	Explicit versus implicit
Strategy	Rational plan versus muddle through
	Global integrated strategy versus piecemeal (incrementalism) strategy
	Elitist control versus grass-roots control
	Proactive strategy development versus reactive strategy development
Sociotechnical	
Teams	Medical care (disease) delivery versus health (preventive) delivery
	Individual prima donnas versus team play
	Reimbursement (financial) realities versus service needs
	Quality of care versus quantity of care
Organizational structure	Service delivery demands versus discipline (functional) demands
	Quantity of care versus quality of care
	Loosely organized versus tightly organized
	Think and behave matrix (be paradoxical, deal with conflict) versus think and behave linearly (be consistent, avoid conflict)
Organizational processes	Quality of decisions versus commitment to decisions
	Quality of decisions versus time to make decisions
	Commitment to decisions versus time to make decisions
	Error-avoiding control systems versus error-embracing control systems
People	Investment in system versus investment in people
	Innovators encouraged and supported versus doers
	Leaders encouraged and supported versus followers
Emergent networks and processes	One dominant coalition versus multiple (pluralistic) coalitions
	Consensus oriented versus dissension oriented

Source: Compiled by the author.

TABLE 2.4

Importance of Goals as Rated by
Sample of MLK Staff

	Percent Rating as Very Important		
Goal	Overall	Management	Unit 1
To deliver comprehensive family-oriented health care	91 (n = 231)	100 (n = 7)	97 (n = 31)
To help patients deal with their environment and society	67 (n = 231)	76 (n = 7)	68 (n = 31)
To provide training for jobs inside and outside the center for community members	63 (n = 231)	29 (n = 7)	71 (n = 31)
To provide the best quality care even at the cost of less quantity	62 (n = 231)	42 (n = 7)	77 (n = 31)

Source: Compiled by the author.

as guidelines for what should be; to provide a source of legitimacy for people's activities and decisions; to serve as standards for how well individuals, subunits, and the total organization are performing; and to provide insight into the true character of the organization. Without consensus among organization members, these functions are likely to work at cross-purposes, for example, when problems occur in making strategic decisions due to underlying goal differences among the decision makers. As we shall see, MLK is currently facing a time when strategic decisions need to be made, yet there is a lack of goal consensus that could undermine effective strategic decision making.

The important trade-offs for MLK in the mission and strategy formulation area are

1. Striking a balance between high faith in its mission versus a minimal faith in its mission. Too much faith makes the organization inflexible and unable to change. Too little provides no commitment to act.
2. Balancing being proactive versus being reactive in developing strategy. Too much proactivity in the form of trying to anticipate events too far in the future can result in diverting energy and attention away from running the organization in the present. Too little proactivity, or a totally reactive stance, may result in unanticipated changes catching the organization totally unprepared and unable to respond.

3. Balancing elite control of organizational strategy versus grass-roots control. The elite group sometimes has the vision and must generate the organizational energy, thus pushing and pulling in ways the majority would not. On the other hand, grass-roots control can build morale and in some situations develop strategy.

Sociotechnical Arrangements

The sociotechnical component is subdivided into team structure and overall organization structure. The team structure represents the basic service delivery unit at MLK, which is an interdisciplinary health team. The design and structuring of the team involve making trade-offs between medical care (disease-oriented) delivery versus health (preventive) care delivery. This trade-off is particularly difficult for MLK, as the current fee for service health financing system within which MLK functions provides financial incentives for disease-oriented care (by paying for medical procedures to take care of people after they are sick) and disincentives for preventive care). MLK's teams were developed and designed to emphasize preventive care, yet in order to survive they must be financially viable, thus the dilemma. Other team level trade-offs include individual prima donna orientation of many physicians versus a collaborative team work orientation and balancing quality of care versus quantity of care.

The organizational structure provides another set of dilemmas. Because teams are assigned specific, relatively permanent, patient populations to serve, a conflict can arise between which kinds of services are offered by different teams. Variations in service needs can result in conflict over who actually decides what services will be provided and in what manner they should be delivered. This conflict over services puts the disciplines (pediatrics, internal medicine, nursing, and so on) on one side and administration on the other.

On the one hand, the market needs (based on the health consumers) could be emphasized, that is, provide a set of services geared to a particular market. For example, as services change, alter the types of providers on the team; or if the population being served becomes older, then cut back on pediatricians. On the other hand, this kind of program runs counter to the dominant tradition in health organizations, which is for the providers (primarily physicians) to determine what services will be offered with little attention given to market considerations, that is, need for service, within limits the physicians can generate need.

A balance must therefore be struck between how much control to give disciplines and how much the market (patient service needs) in deciding on what services to offer. As shall be seen in Chapter 7, the matrix structure builds this conflict explicitly into the organization with equal weight given to each side.

There are dilemmas at the team level that also reveal themselves at an organizational level, such as emphasis on quality of care versus quantity of care. If quality totally dominates, then it is conceivable to have a system where every single procedure is double-checked and audited. On the other hand, if there is no concern for quality, then there would be no need for such procedures as medical audits, which currently exist at MLK.

The organizational structure must also strike a balance between being too loosely organized, resulting in sloppiness, duplication, and so on, and being too tightly organized, resulting in rigidity and a lack of creativity and innovation. The particular organizational design alternative developed at MLK, the matrix structure, poses management with the problem of thinking and behaving "matrix" (Davis, 1976) (being paradoxical, dealing with conflict) versus thinking and behaving linearly (being consistent and avoiding conflict).

Organizational Processes

In the process component, the focus is on such scales or dilemmas as balancing the quality requirements for decisions versus the time available for making the decision. Another scale is the balance between control systems geared to catching errors that encourages avoiding mistakes versus control systems designed to catch errors and learn from them, thus encouraging risk taking. One end of the scale emphasizes punishing mistakes, the other learning from mistakes (Hrebiniak, 1977).

People and Emergent Networks and Processes

The final two components presented in Table 2.3, people and emergent networks and processes, will be discussed jointly. MLK's development provides a fascinating chronicle of how diverse individuals and networks of people with often competing constituencies and agendas can successfully forge a workable collaboration. During its short ten years of existence, MLK has successfully brought together medical professionals from Montefiore, black and Puerto Rican community members, management school faculty from MIT and Columbia, as well as such diverse professionals as lawyers, anthropologists, and community organizers.

The more common experience in poverty programs, especially in the OEO ventures, was that such mixtures of people created a situation leading to spontaneous combustion, often destroying the organization. There were conflicts at MLK among all of these diverse elements, but in all cases conflicts were managed and negotiated, leaving MLK without any serious organizational scars. In fact, many of the conflicts led to valuable new developments.

The force behind the process of successfully linking together people and networks was Harold Wise. Deloris Smith, current director of MLK, then one of the key community members involved with MLK, viewed Dr. Wise in the following terms: "I remember thinking at the meeting that I thought Harold was crazy. And I said to myself, 'He looks like a little kid. They are never going to let that kid do anything. He is just dreaming.'" (Personal interview, 1976.)

Dr. Wise was charismatic, that is, he could "exercise diffuse and intense influence over the normative orientations of other actors" (Etzioni, 1961, p. 203). The early days at MLK were ones that relied on normative power requiring moral involvement and hence a greater need to rely on the use of charisma (Etzioni, 1961, p. 210). As MLK developed these needs shifted and charisma embodied in the person of a leader became less functional. The critical point is that Wise was capable of injecting his dreams into other people's blood in such a way as to mobilize them so that they would make the dreams come true.

Some of the key trade-offs with respect to people at MLK include how much to invest in the development of the system and how much in the development of people. In the early years a very explicit agenda for the center was job training for community members, which included training individuals to work in health-related jobs outside MLK. Also, MLK invested heavily in training and education of its management group, including release time and expenses for university programs. By 1975 the balance on this scale swung to very little investment in individual development.

Another trade-off for MLK to manage has been how much to encourage innovators and entrepreneurs versus how much to encourage doers. This is a dilemma because many of the MLK innovators are not the best workers for carrying out routine day-to-day work. A related but distinct trade-off is determining the balance between the number of leaders and the number of followers needed in the organization.

The trade-offs with regard to emergent networks and processes include whether one dominant coalition is better than multiple coalitions. In the former, one dominant group can guide the organization, while in the latter multiple groups must negotiate an order. Related to this issue is the balance between an organization with a high degree of consensus on issues versus one with a great deal of dissension (Weick, 1969). As we shall see, depending on such conditions as environmental uncertainty and the organization's phase of develoment, the balance is appropriately set at different positions for these two scales (Tichy, 1978).

Chapter 3 examines MLK's strategy in three domains—health, environment, and administration—over the ten years of its existence.

3

MISSION, STRATEGY, AND
OBJECTIVES

. . . Good managers don't make policy decisions . . . rather, they give their organizations a sense of direction, and they are masters of developing opportunities. . . . the successful general manager does not spell out detailed objectives for his organizations . . . he seldom makes forthright statements of policy . . . he is an opportunist, and he tends to muddle through problems—although he muddles with a purpose.
Edward Wrapp, "Good Managers Don't Make Policy Decisions," *Harvard Business Review* 45, no. 5 (1967): 91.

TRADE-OFFS

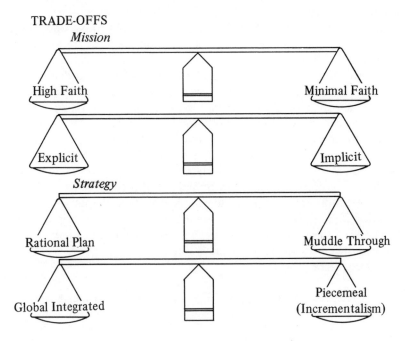

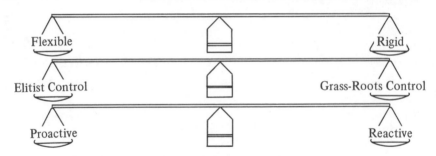

STRATEGIC DECISION MAKING
AND STRATEGY AT MLK

The model presented in Chapter 2 includes a component labeled "mission, strategy, and objectives." As noted in that chapter, all organizations have a mission, a raison d'etre, a strategy. These are guidelines that determine its future and objectives, albeit often not explicit and not agreed on by organization members. Much of the management literature argues for systematic strategic planning, defined as "the determination of the basic long term goals and objectives of an enterprise, and the adoption of course of action and allocation of resources necessary for carrying out those goals" (Chandler, 1962, p. 19).

The normative prescription calls for organizational strategy that is explicit, developed consciously and purposefully, and in advance. As will be demonstrated in this chapter, such a view of organizational strategy is greatly limiting and empirically unrealistic (Braybrooke and Linblom, 1963). Most organizations incorporate a mixture of what Henry Mintzberg (1976a) labels "intended" strategies and "realized" strategies.

Organizations exhibit strategies by virtue of the fact that a series of decisions related to some important aspect of the organization reflects consistency over time without the organization ever having consciously and in advance developed an "intended" strategy. This became the pattern for a number of strategies that MLK followed during its ten-year history, including the pattern of decisions leading to the community management system, the types of health services offered, and the mix of health professionals assigned to primary health care teams.

Therefore, the term "strategy" used in this chapter includes both intended and realized strategy. It is defined as "a pattern in a stream of decisions." In some cases the strategy is intended; in other cases it is realized. The position taken in analyzing stratgegy at MLK is reflected in Mintzberg's statement:

A strategy is not a fixed plan, nor does it change systematically at pre-arranged times at the will of management; the dichotomy between strategy formulation and strategy implementation is a false one because it ignores the learning process that often takes place after an intended strategy is conceived. Indeed, the very word "formulation" is misleading, since what we commonly refer to as strategies may consist of organizational patterns that were not completely developed consciously and deliberately. Even the edict that strategy follows structure misleads, because it ignores the influence that bureaucratic momentum has on strategy formation. The aggressive, proactive strategy maker—the hero of virtually all the normative literature—can sometimes do much more harm than the careful, reactive one. . . . And making strategy explicit in an uncertain environment with an aggressive bureaucracy can do great harm to an organization. . . . (1976a, p. 22)

The important scales in the area of mission and strategy are shown at the beginning of the chapter. In each case, the balance struck brings about the kinds of trade-offs implied in Mintzberg's quote. The analysis of MLK strategy traces the relative weighting of these scales at different points during the last ten years. Chapter 9 ends with a set of recommendations for rebalancing the scales. The recommendations run counter to Wrapp's (1967) advice as well as to Mintzberg's (1976a) warning about normative models. The recommendations are made nevertheless because the conditions appear ripe at MLK for some normative strategic planning prescriptions to begin to function.

CONCEPTS FOR ANALYZING MLK STRATEGY

Organizational strategic decision making entails the dynamic interplay of three factors: organizational environment—its degree of complexity, stability, and uncertainty; organizational momentum—the push by the operating system for stability and the pressure to minimize uncertainty; and organizational leadership—whose role it is to mediate between the environmental constraints and opportunities and the bureaucratic momentum.

As previously indicated, organizations vary greatly and at different times in their own development in how systematically and consciously they make strategic decisions, regardless of the way in which they take place. In the case of MLK, it will be shown that the relative influence of each set of factors varied considerably during different phases of the organization's development, as did the mode by which the leadership made strategic decisions.

Strategy formation is assumed to reflect the organization's attempt via decisions made by the leadership (often referred to as the dominant coalition, those organization members who are able to control the allocation of resources) to maintain control and deal with uncertainty (Thompson, 1967). Uncertainty can be created by events in the environment and/or internal problems. For example, MLK currently faces problems as a result of registered patients moving out of the neighborhood. This is upsetting the equilibrium and requiring the organization to respond strategically. In another situation, there is uncertainty regarding federal funding of neighborhood health centers.

Uncertainty requiring strategic responses can originate both in the environment, as in the above two examles, or within the organization itself, such as when there is trouble between nurse practitioners and pediatricians. In the latter case, the external and internal are interrelated. Leadership has the role of mediating those forces and either consciously or unconsciously coping with the pressures.

Mintzberg (1976a) identified three basic modes of decision making that will be used in the MLK analysis: the entrepreneurial mode—"where a powerful leader makes bold, risky decisions toward realization of his vision of the future"; the planning mode—in which the process is "highly ordered, neatly integrated with strategies determined on schedule by a purposeful organization with explicit goals"; and the adaptive mode— characterized as one in which "multiple decision makers have conflicting goals, bargain among themselves to produce a stream of incremental, disjointed decisions."

In addition to decision-making modes, Mintzberg (1976a) developed a set of terms to characterize aspects of strategic change. These are used in the MLK analysis and include: continuity—strategies are already established and remain unchanged; limbo—the organization hesitates to make strategic decisions; flux—no important consistencies and decision streams seem evident; incremental change—new strategies formed gradually; piecemeal change—one strategy changes quickly while another remains stable; and global change—many strategies change quickly and in unison.

The MLK strategies to be discussed are separated into three major themes: service strategy—decisions about the types of health services to be provided; administrative strategy—considerations on how to manage and organize the health center; and community involvement—relationship of the center to the community and how community input and control are to be integrated into operations.

The remainder of this chapter will establish perspectives designed to help the reader understand what the organizational strategies were and how these strategies came to be. The following section provides a brief chronological overvew of strategy in each of these areas during the last ten years. The section is subdivided into three sections, each referring to a dominant mode of strategy decision making.

Table 3.1

Summary of Shifts in Mission and Strategy Scales

| | Phases | | | | | | | |
| | I Entrepreneurial Mode | | | | II Planning Mode | | III Adaptive Mode | IV Planning Mode |
	Early 1966 Flux	Late 1966 Global Change	1966–69 Start-up and Continuity	1969 Piecemeal Change	1970 Global Change	1971–73 Continuity	1974–76 Limbo and Flux	Recommendations
Mission								
Degree of faith in	High	High	High	Moderate	High	High	Moderate	High
Degree of explicit/ implicit	Implicit	Explicit	Moderately explicit	Moderately explicit	Explicit	Explicit	Moderately implicit	Explicit
Strategy								
Degree of rational/ muddle	Muddle	Muddle	Muddle	Muddle	Rational	Rational	Muddle	Rational
Degree of global/ piecemeal change	Piecemeal	Global	Moderately global	Piecemeal	Global	Global	Piecemeal	Global
Degree of flexible/ rigid	Flexible	Flexible	Flexible	Flexible	Flexible	Rigid	Moderately rigid	Flexible
Degree of elite/ grass-roots control	Elite	Elite, some grass roots	Elite with moderate grass roots	Elite	Elite	Elite	Elite	Elite with moderate grass roots
Degree of proactive/ reactive	Proactive	Proactive	Proactive	Reactive	Proactive	Proactive	Reactive	Proactive

Source: Compiled by the author.

Table 3.1 summarizes how the scales shifted over time as MLK passed through its various phases of development. MLK's development is divided into three major phases indicating the dominant decision-making mode during that period: entrepreneurial mode from 1966 to 1970, the planning mode from 1970 to 1974, and the adaptive mode from 1974 through the present. Within each of these categories, subphases are identified using Mintzberg's terms. These subphase titles describe how strategies changed at that particular point in time.

A BRIEF HISTORY OF MLK STRATEGY

I: Entrepreneurial Mode

Strategic decision making during the early years at MLK was dominated by Dr. Wise's charismatic style. He set the stage and was joined shortly by a core of highly committed, ideologically driven colleagues who dominated the organization until 1970.

Early 1966: Flux

Dr. George Silver, a physician at Montefiore who had run an innovative family maintenance home care program (Silver, 1963), conceived the idea of a neighborhood health center in the early 1960s as a way of improving health care in the Bronx. Harold Wise became director of ambulatory care at Morrisania, a hospital affiliated with Montefiore, which served a large number of residents in the South Bronx. In many respects, the MLK project was an outcome of the sense of shock and outrage Wise experienced at Morrisania. He said:

> I couldn't believe it . . . the place was a slaughterhouse. I had been critical of Kaiser but that was a paradise compared to what I found at Morrisania. I remember thinking at the time: 40 to 50 million people in this country are receiving care like this. As a Canadian, I was poorly prepared to deal with this reality. Canada has had programs of social medicine for many years. (Personal interview, 1974.)

Dr. Silver also had been appalled at the conditions at Morrisania, and had written a proposal for team-delivered care utilizing a doctor, a public health nurse who would function as team leader, and a social worker. The proposal was never funded. In 1966, under the favorable climate of OEO funding and with Dr. Silver then in Washington as a deputy at OEO, Dr. Wise revised Dr. Silver's proposal, substituting family health worker for social worker.

Even though things were in flux owing to the lack of a strategy at this point, there were the beginnings of strategic themes in each of the three domains. In the service area, it was clear that there was a commitment to provide comprehensive health care. In the administrative area, a clear commitment existed for team organization and delivery of care. Finally, community involvement was initially thought of in terms of employing indigenous health workers. Nevertheless, there was much disagreement about specific means and goals in all three domains.

Decisions during this period were largely determined by ideology and value judgments. The environment was generous and supportive and no bureaucratic momentum had built up as yet.

A glance at Table 3.1 indicates that the mission of MLK was not yet clearly explicit at this time, even though there was high faith in a set of values and in a vague image held by Harold Wise and other core staff. The strategy scales were tilted toward a muddling mode, piecemeal change, flexible strategy with elite control and a proactive orientation.

Global Change: Late 1966

Once the health center was funded, the scales shifted. Most notable was that the mission became more explicit and the strategic changes became more global with greater grass-roots involvement, although it was still clearly elitist dominated. Wise was committed to provide comprehensive primary care services, including home visits, preventive care, and care that treated psychosocial health problems. Administratively, the central organizing theme was care delivered by interdisciplinary teams in which the physician would not dominate but would collaborate. The community strategy was stated as "to involve, and where possible, to employ . . . neighborhood inhabitants in the organization, policy planning, operation and provision of services" (MLK, 1971, p. 2).

There were a number of reasons for this dedication to community involvement. First, OEO guidelines necessitated some acknowledgment of community input. Second, Wise had a commitment to such involvement, based on his experience with consumer input in a health center in Saskatchewan, Canada. Nowhere in Wise's original proposal, however, were there any concrete plans on how to implement community involvement, other than to provide training, jobs, and to create some sort of community advisory board. Wise had a relatively clear idea of goals for community and service but not for administration.

1966–69: Start-up and Continuity

Within two months after funding, Wise had selected a core group of professionals whose duty it was to move into the community as organizers. The group included Dr. William Lloyd, a physician and associate of Dr. Wise at Montefiore; Stella Zahn, director of training; Harriet Bogard, a young attorney and community organizer; Roy Kurahara, community organizer; and Ronald Brooke, director of research.

In short order, this handful of gifted "outsiders" was able to mobilize the community around the proposed center. Apartment meetings were held at the project. Ronald Brooke, a research expert, was engaged in a community health survey that was strategically linked with Kurahara's community organizing efforts. Ms. Zahn set up her training shop in a basement apartment in the project, and Ms. Bogard began classes on health advocacy, teaching community members how to obtain their legal rights. A community involvement strategy began to unfold. Eventually, the strategy became one based on an alliance between the professional outsiders who gained the trust of key community members and who viewed the center as a source for jobs.

The health survey and community organizing laid the groundwork for Ms. Zahn to implement what became one of OEO's most successful training programs. Ms. Zahn is a highly competent realist who appears to have had little use for some of the more idealistic training theories that prevailed at OEO at the time. These included the belief that scooping only the cream from the population to supply the staff was a heinous practice. Instead, the OEO theory was that "hard-core" elements should be selected to make up the staff.

Contrary to this theory, the MLK selection process rigorously took only the cream from the pool of candidates, choosing only the high quality candidates who would be able to benefit from the training. A direct result of this decision is that two of the current top managers, Deloris Smith and Kathleen Estrada, came from the original group of candidates. It was this selection and socialization process that eventually brought about community involvement. The promulgated normative standards were commitment to the mission, willingness to work long hours, and ability to take large responsibilities. Although Dr. Wise was supportive and encouraging, he also made a practice of throwing people in over their heads in many situations, and seeing who would sink or swim.

After a year, the smaller of MLK's two locations, the Bathgate Center, opened. It began to operate in a way consistent with the intended service and administrative strategies. There were two health teams providing a wide variety of medical and health-related services, including assistance in medicolegal matters. People on the teams felt a sense of mission to be part of a highly innovative enterprise. Yet, by the end of the 1966–69 start-up period, there was confusion over team roles, about who does what, with whom, when, and so on. And organizational tensions began to occur.

The leadership did not have to manage much with regard to the environment because OEO provided generous financial support with few constraints. Montefiore was taking a very protective "hands-off" position. And the community board was a benign force, headed by a woman who was a strong supporter of Wise.

The scales remained balanced at about the same points throughout this period. Two changed slightly. The mission became less explicit as more individuals joined the organization. These new members brought with them slightly different agendas about what MLK should be trying to accomplish. Lack of a mechanism for explicitly working toward defining a common organization mission resulted in it becoming less explicit. Also, the scale with global strategic changes characteristic of the pre-start-up days on one side was beginning to tilt toward more piecemeal strategic changes on the other side.

1969: Piecemeal Change

This phase marked the turning point for MLK, both in regard to community strategy and administrative strategy. The country's enthusiasm for the Great Society with its War on Poverty was waning. Community political maneuvering and patronage began to exert new pressures on MLK through the board. Internal pressures were also growing because of a fourfold increase in size with the opening of a branch of the center on Third Avenue. (This branch was staffed by six teams, increasing MLK's size from two to eight teams.) These new pressures ultimately brought on a total reorganization and a shift toward more formalized community control via a community management system.

Leadership was subjected to considerable stress during this period, culminating with Wise taking a year's leave to collect his thoughts and back off from the frustration generated in the organization with his charismatic style.

The many strategic shifts that took effect during this phase were accomplished more or less unconsciously and in a piecemeal fashion. All three strategic domains can be characterized as exhibiting entrepreneurial modes of decision making. By the end of this phase, however, things were not working well. The shift away from community control via an external board, which emerged in response to external problems, brought problems. Furthermore, there were also a variety of administrative changes made by Dr. David Kindig, the new medical director, undertaken to systematize the sloppier aspects of the MLK administration. All of these changes, however, were occurring as separate, nonintegrated responses.

By the end of this phase most of the scales, as indicated in Table 3.1, were in new positions. The faith in MLK's mission was moderate as the organization's growth inevitably added people to the staff who were less ideologically committed to the mission of the organization and more personally instrumentally oriented. The mission continued to become less clearly articulated and explicit.

The strategic decision-making style was to muddle through in a piecemeal fashion with the elite group reacting to changes in the environment as well as waiting for things to go wrong in the organization before acting.

II: The Planning Mode

1970: Global Changes

The external environment continued quite placid during this phase. OEO still provided good financial support with minimal emphasis on productivity. Montefiore's stance continued to be supportive and hands-off. An Intern and Residency Program in Social Medicine at Montefiore, which was to become an important source of physician staff for MLK, was established by Dr. Wise. But, at the same time, there was a worsening of relationships with the community board. The MLK response was a shift toward developing a community management system, coupled with trying to keep the community board at arms-length.

The real pressure and uncertainty, however, came from internal administrative confusion and frustration. Several new and major strategic decisions were made during this period. The pressure was of sufficient intensity for Dr. Wise to seek outside help, which was when Richard Beckhard was brought in from the Sloan School of Management at MIT.

Beckhard brought management and organization design expertise to MLK, thus providing the group with new models for dealing with their problems. Professor Beckhard worked with the top management and the community heirs apparent, Deloris Smith and Sonia Valdez, in clarifying the MLK mission and priorities in all three domains—service, administration, and community. Once this was done, it was clear to Beckhard that the MLK structure and management was ineffective. It no longer provided effective team-oriented health care with maximum community and worker involvement and control.

Beckhard filled these administrative gaps by initiating an alternative organizational design and other managerial mechanisms. Thus MLK management shifted to a rational planning mode. The resulting strategic decisions were the reorganization of MLK to a matrix type of structure (discussed in detail in Chapter 7); team development work carried out by a group of MIT consultants under the direction of Dr. Irwin Rubin (see Chapter 6); and a carefully worked out strategic plan for developing a community management system (see Chapter 4).

Dr. Wise left MLK permanently once the global strategic change was completed.

1971–73: Continuity

This was the consolidation phase, with the strategies formulated in the previous stage being carried out. The changes appeared to follow a rather typical scenario: from charismatic leadership, to routinization of charisma, to bureaucracy (Weber, 1964; Etzioni, 1961). Strategic plans had been formulated to allow for a more efficient organization as well as for implementing a viable community management system. Largely under the forceful leadership of Dr. Edward Martin, the new director of health services, these plans were promulgated. Dr. Martin was relentless in his pursuit of having MLK follow the rules and pull its own financial weight, while at the same time providing quality care. Martin anticipated the gradual decline in federal support, as well as the destructive impact of hostile political and social attitudes toward OEO projects.

III: Adaptive Mode

1974–76: Limbo and Flux

The global strategic plans developed in 1971 came to fruition in 1974. MLK was beginning to deliver the kind of service intended. Interdisciplinary health teams were functioning in a matrix type of structure. A community management system was in place and operating. But other things were changing, especially in the external environment. Pressure for increased financial viability began mounting from both HEW and Montefiore. Training funds were cut.

Initially, the organizational strategy slipped into limbo. Strategic decisions were made slowly. However, as environmental pressure mounted, strategy formulation moved into flux. No decision streams were evident. In the clinical service area, new programs, such as a needed hypertension program, were inadequately implemented. Pressure for quantity was affecting quality as evidenced by deterioration of interaction at team conferences.

Administratively, the matrix structure was being subverted by not giving equal weight to service quality requirements and quantity requirements. In fact, most of the stress began to be placed on the quantity side of the matrix. The community control plan, whose task it was to create a board with responsibility over the grant, became stalled. Attempts by the management group to formulate future plans were started in 1975 but never carried out. Pressure was mounting both from the environment and internally for yet another global organizational change. In the meantime, the overall situation continued in flux. There was an anxious, disjointed search for solutions to pressing problems. The old integrated strategy was disintegrating. But no clear new strategies had emerged by the beginning of 1977.

The final phase of MLK's development has brought the scales to a new state of balance. The faith in the mission is now only moderate and the mission is moderately implicit. Strategic decisions are characterized by muddling, piecemeal, moderately rigid, elite control, and, to date, a relatively reactive stance. There are signs of change, as in early 1977 the leadership group had begun to address the external and internal sources of uncertainty. Chapter 9 presents a plan for rebalancing the MLK mission and strategy scales.

4

**THE COMMUNITY
MANAGEMENT SYSTEM**
Noel Tichy
with June Taylor

Did the War on Poverty increase the participation of the poor? Judging from such projects as Mobilization for Youth, it would seem that the millions of dollars spent in the name of the poor largely benefited the middle class, supplying employment to thousands of professional elites, be they black, Spanish-speaking, or white (Helfgot, 1974).

MLK is the exception.

TRADE-OFFS

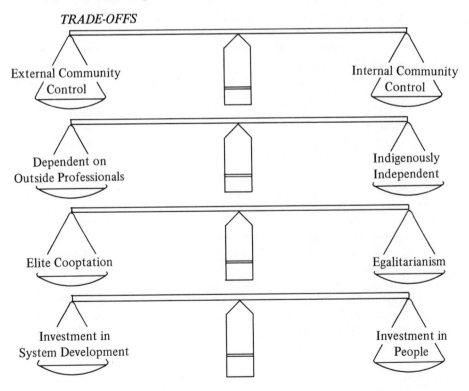

External Community Control — Internal Community Control

Dependent on Outside Professionals — Indigenously Independent

Elite Cooptation — Egalitarianism

Investment in System Development — Investment in People

INTRODUCTION

The relationship of federally sponsored War on Poverty organizations to their environments has been fraught with conflict and contradictions. The managerial and organizational dilemmas of organizations such as MLK are characterized by the following scales that need balancing:

1. The degree of external versus internal community control. External control is generally exercised through some type of legal board mechanism, whereas internal community control can be exercised by employing community residents, including making them managers.
2. Degree of dependence on outside professionals versus indigenous independence. In medical organizations requiring physicians and nurses, poverty communities must import outside professionals. A managerial and organizational dilemma is how dependent the organization becomes on the outside professionals.
3. Degree of elite cooptation versus radical egalitarianism. Critics on the left criticize the efforts of liberal reformers as examples of "imperialist" cooptation where the best community members are coopted via jobs into the system and in turn act no differently than outsiders in ignoring and being unresponsive to the needs of the poverty community. The degree to which this is true and the degree to which a more radical egalitarian institution is created are dilemmas MLK faced throughout its development. Cooptation has long been a viable method for an organization to cope with elements in its environment. James Thompson and William McEwen define cooptation as a method by which an organization ". . . adjusts to the pressure of specific centers of power within a community . . . through the . . . process of absorbing new elements into the leadership or policy determining structure of an organization as a means of averting threats to its stability or existence" (1958, p. 27).
4. Degree of investment in system development versus investment in people. Most organizations face this dilemma. However, the OEO-sponsored organizations had to deal with this as a central issue due to the fact that one of the goals of the War on Poverty was community participation through jobs, and there were plenty of job training funds available. The managerial dilemma is to determine the appropriate investment, as there were times when MLK was investing far more in developing people than in the system, including training many more people for health jobs than could be absorbed by MLK.

These four scales changed their balances over the three major phases of MLK's development (see Table 4.1). This development is traced in this chapter.

COMMUNITY PARTICIPATION AND COMMUNITY CONTROL

Community participation emerged as a major policy issue in the War on Poverty; the Economic Opportunity Act of 1964 required that antipoverty programs be carried out with "maximum feasible participation" of the residents of the communities involved. From its first formal promulgation, the concept was controversial (Moynihan, 1969; Rubin, 1969). The term was also highly ambiguous and variously defined according to the exigencies of the situation. In retrospect, it appears that neither its advocates, its opponents, nor indeed OEO had a clear understanding of the meaning of the term.

Community participation became a significant issue in the health field because of the focal position of neighborhood health centers in the War on Poverty. Health became politicized and the health centers became a social movement (Hollister, Kramer, and Bellin, 1974). Previously in the United States, health delivery had been considered the responsibility of physicians and other professionals; past efforts at reform in the health field were professionally oriented and had generally focused on improving the education, responsibility, and accountability of physicians. The introduction of community participation into the health field was a distinctly new development. A major point of confusion was the lack of clear distinction between community participation and community control.

H.J. Geiger (1974) noted that these two terms have not been clearly understood by the participants, and that many of the problems in the neighborhood health centers are related to this lack of comprehension. Paul Torrens (1971) related community participation to issues of authority and power. He noted that there is administrative uncertainty in neighborhood health centers because the real center of authority has not been determined. E. Feinhold (1970) has discussed the ambiguity regarding the relationship of participation to power in the context of politics and the management of conflict:

> Precisely what was meant by community participation was never clearly defined by OEO, in the traditional American method of avoiding conflict through ambiguity. The problem with this method is that it avoids conflict on one level only to create it at another (p. 113).

TABLE 4.1

Community Control Scales

	Phases of MLK's Development		
	Phase I: 1966–70	Phase II: 1970–74	Phase III: 1974–Present
Degree of external versus internal community control	External Moderate	Internal Moderate	Internal Moderate
Degree of dependence on outside professionals versus indigenous independence	High dependence on outside professionals	High dependence on outside professionals	Moderate indigenous independence
Degree of elite cooptation versus radical egalitarianism	High degree of elite cooptation	Moderate degree of elite cooptation	Low degree of elite cooptation
Degree of investment in system versus investment in people	High investment in people	Moderately high investment in people	Low investment in system (none in people)

Source: Compiled by the author.

Definitions of Community Participation and Community Control

In this chapter, the terms "community participation" and "community control" are differentiated. Community participation can range from full control of a center by indigenous representatives, to partial representation as staff members or board members, and all the way to various forms of "symbolic representation," in which minority professionals serve as representatives of the poor (Helfgot, 1974).

For our purposes, community control of an organization refers to the power to make policy and administrative decisions. In our discussion of MLK, we consider the community management system to be a major step in the direction of full community control. "Full" community control entails formal policy-making and managerial control by an indigenous group.

Community control is generally discussed in terms of indigenous participation. Some form of representation is implied. Individuals, in some way representative of the community, participate as clients, staff, or as members of advisory or policy-making bodies. The term "indigenous participation" has been used quite loosely in the literature. Helfgot (1974) has noted that ethnicity is often used as the equivalent of indigenous origins, so that middle-class minority professionals often serve as symbolic representatives of the poor. Therefore, for our purposes, indigenous implies not only ethnicity but also contiguity in class and residence. In the case of MLK, community managers are individuals representative of the community served in all of the above aspects.

Most of the OEO health centers conceived of community participation through a community advisory board. The board was expected to evolve to a point where it would be capable of assuming responsibility over the federal grants that were generally awarded through larger medical centers. The boards would thus evolve from advisory to policy-making bodies. A stipulation to this effect was written into contracts awarded in the mid-1960s.

The terms of participation were ambiguous, however, and the functions of the boards were not clearly defined. In some manner, community participation was expected to lead to community control, during some unspecified time span; this appears to be the policy underlying the ambiguous OEO guidelines. As long as the policy was implicit, it could be accepted by more moderate elements as a form of "gradualism," which to some viewers had distinctly neocolonial overtones. On the other hand, more radical reformers could interpret the strategy as one of "putting pressure on the system."

Although most centers emphasized the hiring and training of indigenous staff for paraprofessional "new careers" jobs, there was, on the whole, very little effort to move such paraprofessionals into administrative and managerial positions. This would have been one way to increase community control within the center.

The relationship between the internal and external aspects of community control is largely unexplored. In a recent collection of articles on neighborhood health centers (Hollister, Kramer, and Bellin, 1974), the editors commented that most discussions of community participation have overlooked the internal dimension. MLK is cited as an example of a center that has vigorously pursued a policy of worker participation while "eschewing the consumer representative route."

Internal Versus External Control

In this section, we will develop a theoretical framework for the analysis of internal versus external community control in neighborhood health centers. Figure 4.1 displays some of the possibilities in two-dimensional framework. Path 1 in Figure 4.1, developing external board control, at the outset does not appear to be a fruitful route leading to full community control. It is difficult for a community board to undergo the necessary training and development while the organization is being managed by outsiders toward whom they feel defensive.

In the MLK model (Path 2 in Figure 4.1) an internal management system is developed before there is a firm commitment to grant policy-making power to the community board. Outside elites come into the community and train an indigenous worker elite to take over the system as managers. This strategy creates organizational stability, as the necessary skills and knowledge are absorbed by the community work force. Then, development takes place on the external dimension (Step C in Figure 4.1).

Another model (Path 3 in Figure 4.1) would involve developing control over both dimensions simultaneously. It is theoretically difficult and as yet untried in the medical field. Its implementation would require large expenditures of training resources and benign internal and external environments. This route ultimately may prove to be the most efficient approach to community control when more is learned from experimental programs such as MLK. At this point, it is premature to advocate it as a model.

MLK pursued several paths in its movement toward community control. Figure 4.1 depicts them as Steps A, B, and C. Step A was along Path 1, which represents initial attempts to implement OEO policy regarding community involvement. There was an ideological commitment made to "hand over the center to the community" in a manner not clearly defined. A board was established during this step. Step B was taken because of failures in Step A. MLK staff and Montefiore refused to hand over financial responsibility to the board on the grounds that it was not competent to handle the reins of a complex health center. As a result, friction began to develop between the MLK board and staff. This was followed by a change in emphasis toward achieving community control via the training of indigenous workers to be future managers. This new policy brought with it a gradual shifting of authority and responsibility from physician-managers to community managers via a "mentor system" of training.

Step C represents the present transition phase, the integration of the community management system with the establishment of a policy-making board that will control the grant monies. It is a movement toward full community control along the external dimension.

MLK's movement toward community control involved use of all of the following strategies. We will discuss their employment by MLK and

FIGURE 4.1

Paths to Full Community Control

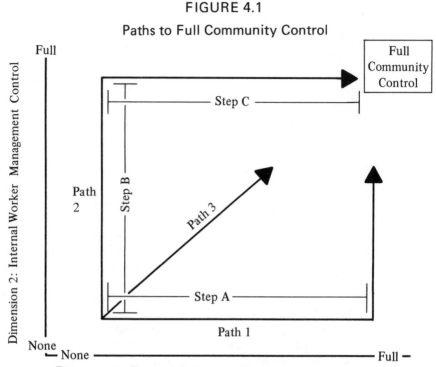

Dimension 1: External Community Board Control

Source: Compiled by the author.

the consequent policy implications for other health organizations. And we will consider the effectiveness of the various strategies in achieving community control. A major concern will be the extent to which the MLK experience can be generalized.

A. External Control Strategies
1. Community scouting and organizing networks. These solicit information about community residents' needs and desires for the health center and the kinds of services delivered, establishing a network of interested and involved community residents.
2. Community advisory board. Establishing a board made up of representatives of the community in terms of ethnicity, class, and residence, either appointed or elected. The board provides advice and informational input to the health center's management.
3. Consumers assigned to one team for all health care. Patients

are assigned to one team of health providers. This increased involvement with a team provides them with greater potential influence over the care they receive.

4. Consumer advocate programs. The health center provides resources for aiding the health consumer. This includes a patient's bill of rights, mechanisms for handling complaints, specific health center personnel assigned to represent consumer interests, and so on.

5. Full community board control. Establishing a community board that has full financial and policy-making control of the health center.

B. Internal Control Strategies

1. Recruitment. Recruitment strategies can aim at trying to map community participation along three dimensions: ethnicity, social class, and race. There are three levels of personnel within the organization: professional, nonprofessional, and administrative-managerial. It is only possible to match some dimensions of community with some levels of personnel, that is, there are no poor physicians.

2. Team structure. Internal work control is enhanced by the team approach to health care delivery in which nonprofessionals and paraprofessionals participate in decision-making and health care activities that are traditionally controlled by professional physicians and nurses.

3. Unit manager system. Creating an administrative structure not controlled by medical professionals and staffed by indigenous individuals; this is a step toward greater internal community control.

4. Training and upward mobility for staff. The existence of training programs that enable staff to acquire new skills so as to be able to move up in the organization. This includes providing opportunities for staff to move from nonprofessional worker status to administrative-management status.

5. Staff council. The establishment of a representative group of workers to provide input into management and policy making of the health center.

6. Mentor relationships. The establishment of mentor relationships for socializing and training community staff to take over important administrative-management positions.

7. Union support. The fostering of union support to encourage staff upgrading and mobility into supervisory and managerial roles.

8. Organization development. The involvement of outside

consultants for aiding in the management and organization improvement activities.

9. Community management system. Long-range plan for having almost all administrative and management functions carried out by indigenous staff.

MLK's movement toward community control utilized all of the above strategies. In the following section, we will discuss the use of these strategies by MLK in the course of its development. In the remainder of this chapter there will be a discussion of the development of the community management system. In Chapter 5 we will consider the community board and its development and dilemmas.

OVERVIEW OF DEVELOPMENT OF COMMUNITY MANAGEMENT SYSTEM

Figure 4.2 summarizes the career paths of the five top managers at MLK. The cylinder also provides a model of the organization. It includes the departments, organizational levels, and the degree of centralization of the positions. The top positions are all located at the nucleus of the organization. Each position has responsibility over a major functional area. The project director has overall operational responsibility.

The vertical lines extending from the boxes listing current top-level positions show the upward path pursued by the five top managers from earlier positions. For example, the current project director started as a family health worker, became a trainer, and moved up to assistant to the director before she was named deputy project director. Along the way she participated in two formal educational programs: a Lehman College, City University of New York, medical service administrator work-study program and a University of Michigan master of public health program, also a work-study program. Not shown are the mentor training relationships that played another significant role in developing this group (see Table 4.2).

HUMAN IMPLICATIONS IN IMPLEMENTING COMMUNITY CONTROL

MLK's history can be divided into three phases: start-up and early operation (1966–70), transition (1970–73), and community management (1974 to the present). These phases are represented on Table 4.3 along with the strategies for both internal and external control associated with

FIGURE 4.2

Community Managers' Careers

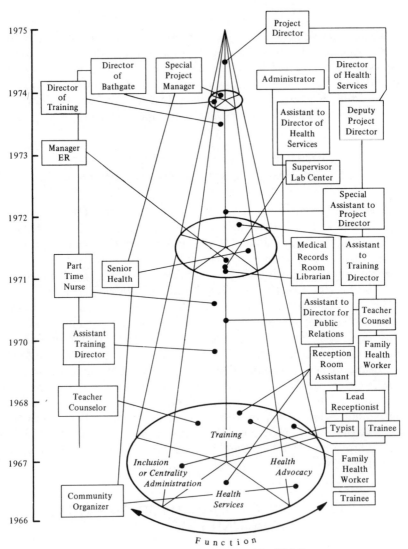

Career Path Development of Key MLK Managers.

Source: Noel Tichy and June Taylor, "Community Control of Health Services," *Health Education Monographs* 4, no. 2 (Summer 1976): 115. (After Edgar Schein, "The Individual, the Organization and the Career: A Conceptual Scheme," *Journal of Applied Behavioral Science* (1971): 401–26.

TABLE 4.2

Training Received by Five Key MLK Managers

Project Director	Director of Health Services	Director of Bathgate Center	Administrator	Special Project Director
1966–Trained as family health worker				No formal program
1969–Lehman College work-study medical service administrator bachelors program (one year)	1969–Correspondence training to receive accreditation for medical records librarian	1969–Public health nurse at start, took 1969–71 to become an anesthetist	1969–Lehman College work-study medical service administrator bachelors program (completed 1973)	
1973–University of Michigan MPA program (completed 1975)				

Note: Key managers also attend relevant professional conferences and participate in management and organization development workshops.

Source: Noel Tichy and June Taylor, "Community Control of Health Services," *Health Education Monographs* 4, no. 2 (Summer 1976): 111.

each phase. We will discuss the use of these strategies by MLK and the policy implications for other health organizations. And the effectiveness of the various strategies in achieving the goal of community control will be considered.

Phase I (1966–70)

The center was founded in 1966, when the establishment of community health centers was taking on the character of a social movement. Community control was always an ideological component of the MLK project.

In 1966, under the favorable climate of OEO funding, Wise wrote a proposal for a consumer-oriented community health center. The proposal

TABLE 4.3

MLK's Strategies for Internal and External Community Control

Phases	Strategies for Internal Community Control	Strategies for External Community Control
I. Start-up and early opera-ation (1968–70)	Recruitment of staff Team structure Training of community members	Scouting community, estab-lishing organizing networks Establishing a community advisory board
II. Transition	Continued staff recruitment Creation of staff council Union support of management Organization development Reorganization plan and plan for community management Mentor relationships Training resources Availability of upward mobility	Advisory board control post-poned. Consumer advocacy programs Patients (consumers) assigned to teams with accountability
III. Community management (1974–75)	Community management system	Phased plan for community board takeover

Source: Noel Tichy and June Taylor, "Community Control of Health Services: Dr. Martin Luther King, Jr. Health Center. Community Management System," *Health Education Monograph* 4, no. 2 (1976): 118.

was supported by Montefiore. The proposal contained basic concepts that have been sustained throughout MLK's history: consumer participation in health care collaborative teams, a strong human rights orientation, and a concern with the social, psychological, and ecological aspects of health. The proposal espoused a strong ideological commitment to egalitarian values in health delivery. Terms such as "mobilization" of the community and "involvement" of the community were used.

During the first year, the project had the pattern of a social movement. There was a central charismatic leader and a core of socially committed professionals who moved into the community as organizers. The exercise of authority was through normative rewards, and in return members' involvement with MLK was moral with high personal commitment to the intrinsic value and mission of the organization (Etzioni, 1961). Community organizing utilized an action-research model. Health needs were surveyed and problems defined in relation to the total community environment.

Organizing networks emerged as an outcome of face-to-face relationships between community residents and the outside organizers. This period set the pattern of the alliance that took shape between professionals and community workers. The two groups were bound together by ties of mutual commitment to the project and by self-interest. The alliance had strong elements of a "social contract" based on reciprocity. The exchange involved mutual support and the pooling of knowledge. This mutuality of interest was critical in the success of the project.

An essential aspect of the social contract was the pledge made by the Montefiore group (both the key administrators and Wise's group) to the effect that the center would eventually be turned over to the community. Although the exact form of this change in jurisdiction was not specified, it is clear that both sides took the commitment literally. One top indigenous manager, Elinor Minor, notes:

> I don't think it would have worked if people like Deloris Smith [the current project director] and Kitty Estrada [the current administrator] had not had the meetings in their apartments. People organizing in the community were used to white outsiders coming in to save them and then going away with things just the same as before. I don't think people would even open their doors to someone making a survey about health. But everyone knew Deloris. She had the respect of everyone in the project as a problem solver, a person who could get things done. If she said they were OK, they were accepted. Everyone started coming to the apartment meetings. (Personal interview, 1974.)

Many of the community residents who were attracted to the program were interested in working at the center. As one MLK manager recalled, "the agenda of the first meetings was jobs." Among the community residents to sponsor the first apartment meetings on the subject of the center were the present director, the administrator, and others who have since become managers. They participated in the first Family Health Worker Training Program. (The Family Health Worker Training Program represents a major contribution on the part of MLK to new health-provider roles. The training was extensive, and the total curriculum is carefully outlined in a booklet distributed by MLK.)

Once the center was in operation, plans were made to turn it over to a policy-making community board. Wise recalls his first commitment to the concept of community control:

> We went around all over the place telling people the center would belong to them. We really believed it. Then Cherkasky [the administrator of Montefiore] made me realize it would not work

immediately or even as a short-term possibility. We just could not do it. The community people simply did not have the skills to run a complex health center at that point. I remember feeling shame-faced about this—having to backtrack. Some of us felt we should resign. (Personal interview, June 1974.)

One of the outcomes of this temporary setback was a stronger commitment on the part of Montefiore to the upgrading of community workers through training. Nonetheless, a specific concept of training for management did not develop until a later stage.

Although the community board was a benign factor during the first two years of the program, conflicts began to develop between board and staff over control of the center and patronage (jobs for family and friends of board members) during the third year. At this point, the major cleavages among the board, the middle-class professional staff, and the community workers began to emerge. Since the community was poor in institutions as well as in other resources, the MLK board became one of the few forums for political activities. It therefore attracted a variety of community activists with various political agendas. One of the major issues on the board was the struggle for power between blacks and Puerto Ricans. Increasingly, the board became weighted toward Puerto Rican power.

The situation within the center was very different as the community workers and the professionals became increasingly concerned with health delivery and less involved with broad political and social problems in the community. Although the majority of the center's workers were black, ethnic conflicts were muted because of cross-cutting ties between blacks and Puerto Ricans, a result of on-the-job camaraderie. There was increasing divergence in the relationships between board members and community workers. Initially, they had held a common point of view. But, as the workers became more technically competent and career oriented, they began to view the board members, who served part time and without pay, as uninformed about health matters and unqualified to make decisions about the center. Furthermore, the workers wanted to cool down ethnic conflict, and regarded the playing out of the Puerto Rican-black struggle on the board as a threat to the center.

It is interesting to note that the traditional pattern of rapidly escalating conflict between professionals and community people did not develop at MLK. The honeymoon lasted longer, and the conflicts were considerably less destructive. Furthermore, the workers tended to support the professional staff and constituted a third power group that prevented polarization along ethnic and class lines.

Toward the end of this first period, there were other significant changes that influenced the development of worker management. Shifts in national mood and government policy influenced MLK's movement from the external to internal dimension of community control. By the end of the 1960s, as previously stated, federal enthusiasm for the Great Society was waning. At the same time, community political maneuvering and political patronage were beginning to exert new pressures. On the federal level, community boards were increasingly viewed as unpredictable and potentially dangerous political entities.

Although OEO policy still formally espoused community participation, there was a new emphasis placed on competence in administering grant monies. Advisory boards were restrained from exerting control over the grant until they were judged to be competent. This meant that authority would remain in the hands of the professionals until some unspecified time. But this did not mitigate community pressures on the professional outsiders.

During this time, other significant internal pressures also built up within the center that led to planning and implementation of the community management system. As previously noted, many of these pressures were of the type associated with the maturing of an organization and had the character of bureaucratization. MLK, in effect, had outgrown the social movement phase and had become an established health institution. There were internal pressures for consolidation, greater productivity, and more effective management; these were reinforced by a gradual, but increasing, federal emphasis on productivity.

A central question was one of authority. Many of the new professional and nonprofessional staff members in the expanded organization had not participated in the social movement phase and regarded their work as "just a job." Moral commitment was becoming an ineffective form of control. Nonetheless, the bureaucratization of the system was at odds with the prevailing egalitarian ethos. A new management directed by white male professional outsiders would not be a solution acceptable to the workers and the community.

During this time, Dr. Wise began to explore worker management as a solution to the problem of running a complex health organization with such an egalitarian ideology. Although he had ideas about worker management, he had few precedents to build on, aside from the small-scale Peckham experiment. In many respects, the community management system was an effective compromise among worker management, egalitarianism, and bureaucracy. It was also a workable response to the failure of moving toward community control via an external board.

The community management system reflected Etzioni's observation that "normative compliance is relatively easy to maintain for short periods of time and for nonroutinized activities; it is difficult to maintain for continuous and long run activities" (1961, p. 294). Thus, it provided MLK with a means for routinization of charisma, which is reflected in a greater use of utilitarian controls (salary and established career avenues are two new rewards most emphasized by Weber, 1946).

Phase II (1970–73)

This stage involved MLK's reorganization and the emergence of a worker management system. The combination of internal and external pressures that had built up during phase I ended for the time being any drive on the part of the MLK staff and key Montefiore administrators toward community control through an external community board. However, community control was still a highly espoused aim of both groups. This commitment and the combination of factors to be discussed below led to the community management system plan and its implementation.

During this phase, a staff council emerged in response to a struggle between the board and the professional managers over the firing of a black administrator. It was organized because staff needed more valid information, and also wanted to influence events and prevent racial problems. Membership on the council was open to anyone who could acquire signatures of nine fellow-workers. The staff council included a number of people who later became top and middle managers. The council had members from the paraprofessional and professional management of MLK. The council became inactive after a while and only reappeared when there was to be a change in management; it did play a role in the apointment of a new management group in 1971. Its inactivity was due to a lack of salient issues and concerns over which staff was willing to invest the necessary time and energy to try to influence.

Another factor paving the way for the community management system plan was the involvement of Richard Beckhard of MIT's Sloan School of Management in the reorganization of MLK.

The actual community management plan grew out of the work of a small group of MLK staff, including top managers and several key workers. One of the early tasks was to clarify the center's goals and priorities. Once this was done, it became clear that the way in which MLK was then structured was inconsistent with combining effective team-oriented health care with maximum community and worker control. The result was the reorganization from a traditional hospital structure (comprising nonoverlapping medical and administration hierarchies) to a structure containing nonphysician managers with line authority over the delivery of care within the unit. Professionals performed strictly medical tasks, but reported to the unit manager for administration.

This new structure was coupled with a new concept that has since been labeled by MLK as the "community management system." A commitment was made in the reorganization to develop unit managers from within MLK and that they would be nonmedical professionals. The transition period was to be a time for training. Key community workers who were slated to become the future directors were to be in training with the physician-managers. These were mentor relationships, which had many of the apprentice aspects of medical residency training.

The board, staff council, and management group were all involved in selecting the new project director and medical director. The two top physicians, the acting project director and director of health services, had job descriptions and agreements that explicitly defined their role as transition people, helping to turn over the agency to a community management system within a period of two years.

Plans formulated for a more efficient organization, as well as for the new community management system, were put into action. Four physicians were fired during this time. In general, it was agreed that legitimate grounds existed for the firings. But it was essentially a show of strength, an "I mean business" message. Symbolically this act demonstrated to many in the community that outside professionals could not get away with exploiting the community. Another example was the shifting of approximately 80 personnel in the span of a few weeks. Other significant changes occurred, including the implementation of new management information systems, the selection and training of middle-level managers, and the development of a top-management group.

The two top physician administrators were of the opinion that the MLK organization had to be as effective as possible before being turned over to community management. The development of a sound organizational structure appeared to them to be as important as the development of the new community managers.

By the end of this phase, the physician-administrators were ready to bow out. The hard-nosed way in which implementation took place had a mixed impact on the organizational culture at MLK. But staff members appeared relieved to know where they stood, and much of the frustration with the lack of structure was alleviated. On the other hand, there was a growing fear of the top. Management became more centralized, controlling, and bureaucratic. It seems clear that some idealism had been sacrificed to expediency.

These activities took place in a changing external environment. By the early 1970s, the policy changes pursued by President Richard Nixon began to be felt. The national mood, too, had shifted and the Great Society enthusiasm appeared to be a thing of the past. This meant that pressures began to be exerted on agencies such as MLK to become more self-sufficient.

Fortunately, Montefiore continued its hands-off, supportive posture toward MLK, enabling it to work out its own problems. The friction with the board, which grew very intense during this phase of MLK's development, was more of an annoyance than an inhibiting factor in the development of the community management system. By this time, key MLK and Montefiore staff members had given up on the board and were keeping it at arms-length so as to minimize its interference in MLK's operation. Eventually the union, Local 1199, sided with MLK management and Montefiore in opposition to the notion that the board should gain control of the grant.

This phase ended with an interesting transition, trial-by-fire, test for the new community management system. In November 1973, there was a citywide strike of Local 1199 health workers. This meant that many of MLK's staff were on strike. The director of health services, Dr. Martin, stayed away during the strike to let the community management group test themselves under fire. The test worked. The center stayed on course, as is attested to by one of the present managers:

> The former director of health services was in California and we had to handle the strike on our own. No one could believe he had left or that the center could go on without him, even today some people think he runs this place from Washington. Anyway, we [the community managers] met every night to plan our strategy. Montefiore was calling every morning asking us: did you do this, did you do that and we told them we had already done it. We knew we could manage the center. (Personal interview, January 1974.)

Shortly after the strike, the acting project director, Dr. William Lloyd, stepped down to become assistant director of health services. The director of health services, Dr. Ed Martin, resigned, and the community management system was in operation.

Phase III (1974–77)

The community management system is now fully operational. There is general agreement that it has proven to be a realistic and effective way to administer a neighborhood health center. In the meantime, there have been new efforts by MLK and Montefiore to develop community control at the external level, and the community management system is under close examination. The staff is testing the top managers. The managers are also testing their own ability to manage. HEW and Montefiore are taking a let's-wait-and-see attitude.

HEW is no longer the never-ending source of funds with a benign posture toward productivity. The funding is exerting pressure toward increased productivity and self-sufficiency. And Montefiore's mood has shifted. It is now ready to work toward a goal of making MLK fiscally and administratively independent. In terms of the greater health community, much attention will be paid to how well MLK functions with its community management system, and whether or not the transition to board control is successful.

Many questions remain unanswered regarding the success of MLK's community management system. Some feel that the testing period will have to provide answers to such questions as Will the new managers be harder and more punitive and authoritarian toward subordinates than medical professionals? What happens when top and middle management are almost totally female?

The center has certainly made an impact on the community. While Dr. Wise's comments are colored by pride in the center, his statements on its sucessful struggle to survive are certainly valid:

> The area had no medical resources and could not have developed them. We had hoped that the community could train its own physicians and be self-sustaining, but this was not possible. I think we developed something like "home rule." We were able to develop some very capable managers. MLK is still a long way from worker-management, but is far ahead of anything else in existence. (Personal interview, 1974.)

Dr. Wise was asked if MLK had been able to raise health delivery in its part of the South Bronx to the level of middle-class medicine. He replied:

> It is much better than middle-class medicine; the entire family is treated by a team which has vastly greater resources than the single practitioner. The team can deal with an enormous area of problems affecting health, including the psychological and social aspects. (Personal interview, 1974.)

MLK appears to be a viable organization. The real question, however, is whether it can continue to be innovative. Some people, such as Wise, fear that much creativity has left the organization. Others fear that if it hasn't it will. The balance between an efficiently run organization and a creative one is delicate. Strains generally develop and need to be managed skillfully. Another question is whether the center's management will become more participatory and will begin to reverse some of the centralizing tendencies of bureaucratization.

The final chapter on the subject of community control will be written if and when the grant is turned over to a new board. A new transition phase started. If the current community management group can successfully handle this transition, which includes setting up management and administrative systems currently handled by Montefiore, then it will have passed one important test. If the new board actually assumes control, what was mere rhetoric in the 1960s will have become reality— first, via an internal management structure and, finally, through an external community management system.

Although MLK is today, in 1977, a viable institution, the future presents many unknowns. Now that community managers are in place, much will depend on the relationships they will be able to establish with funding sources, with the health establishment, and with the board. It is not known if they will be in the position to attract the kind of human and financial resources so readily available to powerful, prestigious Montefiore.

Relationships with the board remain problematic. The strategy of furthering community management while neutralizing the board did not resolve the underlying problems. Rather, it deferred them. The question remains whether the staff and board can develop the kind of working arrangements that can effectively balance inevitable conflicts. The next chapter addresses these issues directly.

It is also important to note that community management, as we have described it, is not immune to overly bureaucratic centralizing tendencies. Indigenous leaders can become just as repressive and unrepresentative as outside elites. But the MLK management system is an important step toward full community control. because the center is directed by persons who understand the community from the inside and can develop health programs that are culturally integrated into the life of the community. Nonetheless, the center has not approached full worker management in which power is even more broadly distributed through every level of the system, as Dr. Wise envisioned.

CONDITIONS SUPPORTING THE DEVELOPMENT OF COMMUNITY MANAGEMENT AT MLK

Community management developed at MLK not only because of the implementation of the strategies discussed previously but also because of the existence of certain special conditions that existed within the center and in its external environment. These conditions were largely present at the beginning and continued to form a supportive base for the center in the course of its development. An attempt will be made to identify elements that can be generalized in planning health policy for other neighborhood health centers.

Value commitment: Throughout the history of MLK, the professionals and the community staff have shared a firm commitment to egalitarian and humanistic values. Although there was little or no agreement in the early stages regarding the implementation of these values, there was a shared ideology that helped provide the impetus toward community management. This value commitment was reflected in the organizational culture.

OEO provision of a supportive environment. In the early phases of MLK's development, federal OEO money was readily available with little pressure for productivity.

Support of a major health institution. Montefiore hospital provided a protective environment with few demands for productivity. This enabled the professional and community staff to learn and innovate without undue fear of making mistakes. OEO and Montefiore support enabled MLK to flourish as a "social laboratory." Because pressures on its structure were minimal during its start-up and growth years, MLK had a better chance to develop its experimental structure.

History of innovativeness. Ideas and creativity were rewarded at MLK, especially in the early phases. Such encouragements provided moral support for discussions among worker management to create a community management system.

Mentor training and support relationships. The Montefiore support of the program was facilitated by a network of professional relationships that had developed in the Department of Social Medicine at the hospital. It is of interest that sponsorship relationships, so characteristic of academic medicine, also developed between Montefiore medical staff and key community workers at MLK. This type of professional-paraprofessional collaboration was a distinctive characteristic of the center.

Staff and union support. MLK has exhibited considerable social solidarity during its development. The staff, which is largely composed of indigenous workers, has continuously supported management. This includes the medical professional managers in the early phases and, more recently, the community managers.

Consumer acceptance. MLK has enjoyed a positive image in the community from the very start. It has been regarded as a good provider of services and as a valuable asset to the community.

Organizational mobility. There was a high degree of vertical and horizontal mobility within MLK during its development. This enabled newly trained personnel to make rapid use of their new skills, and also furnished a major incentive to acquire the necessary training for moving into better positions.

Effective, well-funded training programs. A much higher degre of quality training took place at MLK than at other health centers. There was considerable investment in the transfer of knowledge and skills from upper level personnel to community workers.

Quality of human resources. There were two crucial reasons why the quality of human resources at MLK was so high. First, Dr. Wise was able to attract a core group of professionals with strong dedication to the mission of community-oriented primary health care. A stream of talented professionals passed through MLK and supplied much of the energy and skill for its development. After their job was done, these professionals were willing to give up their power and move on. The second reason for the high quality of human resources was the superior performance level of the community members who worked with MLK in the early stages. The development of these talented individuals in the first stage of MLK's existence created the necessary human resources pool for the community management system's successful implementation.

BALANCING THE COMMUNITY MANAGEMENT SCALES

The trade-offs made by MLK are quite clear. The choice was made, as has been discussed, to give up external community control for internal community control. The next chapter will discuss the external side of the scale and the need for possible future rebalancing. MLK was able to counterweight its dependence on outside professionals with indigenous worker independence. The professionals kept moving in and out of the system.

It is possible to argue that the MLK model is simply a "colonial" model in which outside elite develop a local elite. If this is true, the balance between elite cooptation versus egalitarianism remains tilted toward the elite cooptation side.

Finally, a real balance was struck throughout the early years of MLK's development through 1973 between the practice of investment in people development and in system development. Currently, the tilt is toward system development. There are few in-service training programs and virtually no upward mobility is possible. Unless ways are found to change the tilt of this scale, there will eventually be stagnation of human resources.

5

THE COMMUNITY BOARD

The choice is no longer between having a nonboard, which is what we are having today, by and large, and an effective board. The choice is between a board imposed on an enterprise that is both hostile and inappropriate and a board that is an effective organ of the enterprise and appropriate to its needs (Drucker, 1973, p. 636).

TRADE-OFFS

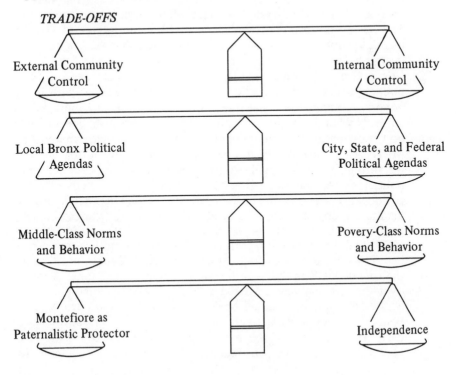

INTRODUCTION

After ten years, MLK appeared on the verge of achieving full community control, as outlined in Chapter 4. As previously stated, the path taken was first to build the internal community management and then to build the external board. The development of a viable community governing board, however, was not yet accomplished by early 1977, even though there was an HEW mandate for the transfer of the governance authority to a community board by January 1978. There was still a question in late 1976 as to whether this would actually occur as the conditions that fostered the development of a community management system did not help foster the development of a community governance board for MLK. The fact that MLK faced greater difficulties in developing the board than in developing the internal management system was in part due to the trade-offs that require balancing in the external control area. These trade-offs are:

1. Degree of external versus internal community control. Although these two are not mutually exclusive, in the early years of MLK's development, the balance was clearly toward internal management control. This helped MLK to minimize disturbances generated by an uncertain environment that were often reflected on the board. The scale may become rebalanced in 1977 due largely to HEW's mandate, not due to a management decision that such a board is desirable.

2. Local Bronx political agendas versus city, state, and federal political agendas. The political agenda in the Bronx, as with many poverty communities, has been focused on which ethnic group controls what institutions. Control of MLK represents considerable power owing to the large number of community people employed by MLK. The organization, therefore, becomes a focus for political infighting between local Puerto Rican and black community politicians. At the same time, MLK has been the focus of other political agendas. As one of the early successful OEO neighborhood health centers, it became a symbol for what the War on Poverty could accomplish in the health field. This meant that OEO and then HEW had a vested interest in seeing it continue to be successful.

    The city and state political agendas focused more on deciding the role of MLK in the overall health system of the Bronx. At times over the last five years, MLK has been viewed by some politicians as the core of a much larger health system for the total Bronx. Such plans were not being actively pursued at the city or state level in early 1977 because of the more pressing financial emergencies in New York. However, if federal money becomes available for developing a larger network of health services in the Bronx, MLK may again be considered the core.

3.   Middle-class norms and behavior versus poverty-class norms and behavior. The exercise of power on boards of public trust organizations is part of the attraction to those who are members. This is true of upper- and middle-class members as well as poverty-class members. However, the norms about appropriate exercise of power are often more subtle among the middle class, whereas the poverty-class members are often found to exercise power in a more direct and often unacceptable manner. For example, it was not unusual in OEO program organizations to find board members intervening directly in line management functioning. There was a time when board members at MLK would come into the center and tell workers how to do their jobs, or board members frequently tried to get friends and family jobs at MLK.

     The difficult balance is to find and/or develop board members from a poverty community who can exercise power in a manner acceptable to the institutions providing the funding and in general accord with the norms and behavior regulating trustee behavior.

4.   Montefiore as paternalistic provider versus independence. This scale is the most difficult to balance, as there is considerable ambivalence on the part of both MLK and Montefiore regarding how it should be balanced. The OEO intention was clearly for MLK to become independent some day, as was the value position of Dr. Wise and the other core group of founders. However, over the years of MLK's development, it became clear that Montefiore was an invaluable resource and protector. The community managers in particular appear to see many advantages in a future that continues to keep MLK as part of the Montefiore system.

The difficulties MLK has faced in developing a board are rather ironic for an organization at the forefront of activities that fulfilled the spirit of the original (Title II) section of the Economic Opportunity Act of 1964, which called for Community Action Programs that were to be ". . . developed, conducted, and administered with the maximum feasible participation of residents of the areas and members of the groups being served."

The one rather clear OEO mandate to which MLK attempted to address itself was the creation of some form of local community governance board. In order to understand why as late as early 1977 the board still had little control or influence over MLK, we must trace several themes back to the start of MLK. Let us first take a brief overview of the community programs and other forms of community participation.

From the start, Harold Wise and his core group of professionals assumed that many of the health problems in the South Bronx were manifestations of inadequate housing, nutrition, and education. As a result, there was always substantial MLK involvement in community development activities. As Wise indicated in 1970:

> The kinds of conditions affecting the state of health of the residents in the area—such as deteriorated buildings, lead based paint, inadequate heating, fire hazards, vermin, poor sanitary conditions, all subvert any provisions of medical service, no matter how good. The patients in the area are numb. The morale of the staff working in such a downward spiral sinks lower and lower. (Wise, 1970)

An example of the importance of community development activities is that Mrs. Sonia Valdez, the director of the center's Community Health Advocacy Department, is a member of top management. The activities carried out by this department and several others have furnished many meaningful ties between the community and MLK. This kind of interaction has reduced the center's need to rely on a board for input and guidance in community matters. The MLK staff, not the community board, have generally been the leaders in promoting community development activities.

Health Advocacy, an Important Community Program

Let us briefly examine the Community Health Advocacy Department's mission: ". . . the creation of a community environment conducive to the provision of the Center's comprehensive, family oriented health services." The specific objectives of the department in 1974 were to improve housing, sanitation, public safety, recreation, education, and specialized services in the community; to impart advocacy skills to community residents and to catalyze cooperative community efforts aimed at bringing about a healthy community; and to define and advocate the legal health rights of people as they relate to direct health services and institutions that affect health (Martin Luther King Health Center, 1970).

The work of the department has included establishing several corporations in collaboration with other neighborhood organizations. The ultimate goal was to solve complex health, housing, and economic development problems. In fact, one organization, the Bathgate Community Housing Development Corporation, was created to sponsor rebuilding and rehabilitation of housing in the area.

Other Community Programs

In addition to the Community Health Advocacy Department, MLK has been extremely active in dealing with patients' rights. In addition to initiating a now widely accepted "patients' rights" pamphlet, MLK invested a great deal of time and effort in the development of a patients' rights manual. The pamphlet became the first step in implementing a patients' rights system at MLK. The entire MLK staff received training related to patients' rights. A system for handling grievances was established and an extensive community outreach effort to distribute the pamphlet personally to each member of all registered families took place. (When this was accomplished in 1970, 5,000 of the 7,000 registered patient family members received a personal copy of the pamphlet.)

The Community Health Advocacy Department and the patients' rights efforts at MLK must be kept in mind when examining the advisory board problems at MLK.

Mixed Motives

Before tracing the history of the advisory board, we will present a brief analysis of the forces at work that kept the advisory board in a state of limbo. As late as 1976, there appeared to be mixed motives on the part of MLK management and on the part of Montefiore management, some pushing toward MLK independence and some pushing toward keeping the status quo. However, by early 1977, the push shifted toward conforming with the HEW mandate for board control by January 1, 1978.

In the past, MLK management and staff enjoyed the following implicit or explicit benefits by staying under the protective arm of Montefiore: they could draw upon the prestige and resources of a large and powerful medical center; as staff members, they received benefits as Montefiore employees (benefit package, easier bank credit, and so on); and they gained a sense of security that allowed them to feel that if MLK got into financial trouble, Montefiore would be there to back them. Whether these benefits were in reality available is not important. What is important is that they were perceived as such.

The negative side of remaining integrated into the Montefiore structure is that the current level of autonomy could easily be reduced. This would certainly happen in the event of financial difficulties. In such a case, it is likely that Montefiore would step in to control and manage operations directly. There is also some perception on the part of the local populace that MLK is merely a tool or token of Montefiore and as a result is not a real community organization.

Montefiore management was not without mixed motives, either. On the side favoring keeping MLK as a vassal instrumentality is the reality that MLK is good public relations for Montefiore. It is a concrete example that Montefiore is doing something for the poor at a time of increasing attacks on Montefiore as functioning only as a middle- and upper-class health provider. Further, MLK is the source of many health innovations, which also accrue credit to Montefiore. Among other things, MLK functions as a training site for Montefiore's social medicine residents in pediatrics, internal medicine, and family practice.

On the negative side, the major force that pushes Montefiore to favor MLK autonomy is the potential financial liability of an organization that is losing patients and facing HEW cutbacks. There are diminishing returns in serving the poor, while the financial risks heighten.

This was the context within which the MLK advisory board operated in 1976. Coupled with the ambiguity and ambivalence that characterized its development since 1966, it was not surprising to see the haphazard status of the board in 1976. The HEW mandate and the active support of Deloris Smith, MLK's director, for board control changed the picture early in 1977 and should lead to full board control by the end of 1977.

HISTORY OF THE BOARD AT MLK

In 1975, a workshop was organized for members of the advisory board, key MLK managers, and one of the deputy directors of Montefiore, Mo Katz. The agenda included plans for transferring the granteeship from Montefiore to an MLK board. This event and many of the activities surrounding it provide a microcosm of the history and some of the issues surrounding the struggle to develop a viable governing board at MLK.

Events Leading Up to the Workshop

The workshop came about as a result of a proposal from the deputy director of MLK to the board in August 1975. At that time, Katz suggested that board members take some time to discuss their position regarding assuming responsibility over the MLK grant. In addition, Katz wanted the board to examine the kind of training individual members would need to equip them to assume greater responsibility in the running of the center. Katz offered the services of an outside consultant (Noel Tichy) to work with the board in conducting the retreat and to help them implement plans that were to be made.

In August 1975, Katz met with the project director, Delores Smith, and the consultant to develop plans for the workshop. At this meeting, Katz stated his desire to help in the development of the board so that it would be able to assume more responsibility. The consultant asked both Smith and Katz to more clearly identify their long-term commitments to the transfer of full granteeship to MLK. Katz supported the turning over of this grant to a board. His only concern was that MLK would get into trouble or become a political football in the process. Smith, on the other hand, was more equivocal. She began by being noncommittal. When questioned about this by the consultant, she stated that she really was not sure that she wanted full granteeship. Ultimately, she indicated that she would like MLK to continue under the Montefiore umbrella.

It was apparent that both Katz and Smith were undergoing an ideological struggle on the subject of the desirability of an independent neighborhood community center. Katz seemed to support the initial policy orientation of OEO, which was to turn the grant over to the center. Ironically, as a former community member who worked her way up through the MLK structure, Smith took a position that would not lead to full community control but would instead keep the center within the Montefiore framework. The seeds for a disagreement between Katz and Smith became apparent. Evidently, Smith at that time saw that more could be gained by a continuing affiliation with Montefiore. At the same time, she felt there was sufficient autonomy and no need for concern about being overly controlled by Montefiore.

MLK Board Workshop, Fall 1975

The conference was scheduled to start at 8:30 p.m. on Friday, October 4, 1975. The expected number for Friday evening was 15. Yet only 6 people were present by 8:15. Mo Katz, who had organized the workshop, was visibly angry. It crystallized his anxiety about the fact that members of the board were irresponsible, childish, and consequently unable to take responsibility for an annual $8 million budget. Friday night's session eventually began with eight people present. This included five board members and three others: Katz, the consultant, and Dr.

William Lloyd (a physician and assistant director of health services of MLK).

Katz began the evening with a general historic overview.

An Overview

Table 5.1 provides a list of some of the key events in the history of the community board. Mr. Katz, Mrs. Lucy Cortez (a community member on the board since the beginning), and Dr. Lloyd collaborated to outline this historic development of MLK and its relationship to the board from their perspectives.

The original board was set up in August 1967. The process for obtaining members for the board included inviting local delegates to a meeting. To be a delegate, one needed 25 signatures from community members. These delegates then met and elected members to the board. Once the board of 21 was selected, orientation meetings were held at Montefiore Hospital.

The early years when Mrs. India Davis was chairman of the board were without incident. The board was very supportive of MLK, and Wise had a very good relationship with Mrs. Davis. Trouble began, however, when an administrator was dismissed. The administrator was incompetent and was fired for good cause. But because Wise took the steps to fire him, the board felt circumvented. Therefore, when the dismissal took effect, the board decided to back the employee. This resulted in a showdown. Wise told the board that an internal administrative matter was involved and that the board had no right to interfere. He went on to refuse to give the board any reason for the administrator's firing. (Part of Dr. Wise's reason was to protect the administrator and not make public all of his gross inadequacies.)

The outcome was that the board and community began to picket the center. Dr. Martin Cherasky, director of Montefiore, intervened. The final agreement led to the firing of the administrator but with severance pay plus tuition for the pursuit of studies in public administration. This incident led to a change in the board and the board chairman. After it, the relationship between the board and the center began to worsen.

The next difficult experience for the board was the receipt of $33,000 a year for its own development and training in 1971. A staff person was hired at $16,000 a year to begin training board members for financial responsibility. This was an unsuccessful episode in the board's development. The board staff person's prime occupation seemed to be to work for political figures. He was not available to work on board matters. As a result, no training or preparation for taking over the grant took place.

TABLE 5.1

Chronology of the MLK Board

Dates	Events
July 25, 1966	OEO grant
June 3, 1967	Opening of Bathgate Center
1967	First board delegates (India Davis, chairman)
September 9, 1968	Main center opens
1969	Second board delegates (Lucy Cortez, chairman)
February 1971	Confrontation over firing of administrator
May 1971	First board training
July 7, 1971	Wise resigns
November 1971	Direct board election
April 1972	New board seated
September 1972	OEO grant to board (first workshop and board staff hired)
August 1973	Transfer of OEO to HEW
October 1973	Second workshop
Sepember 1974	New bylaws
August 1975	Third workshop planned

Source: Compiled by the author.

This phase culminated in a meeting at which representatives of OEO, the total board, and the Montefiore administration met to review the criteria that OEO had given to the board for assuming the grant. The meeting, according to Katz, turned out to be a most embarrassing session. As he tells it, the OEO representative read a list of ten requirements that the board had been asked to meet in order to qualify for granteeship. In each case, the board staff person replied that the requirement had not yet been complied with. The meeting turned out to be an unpleasant experience for all involved. The board had assumed that its staff person had taken care of all ten items. (The OEO requirements included such things as preparation for union negotiation, development of bylaws, planning of board structure, and so on).

The next critical event was the transfer of OEO to HEW. The importance of this event is that HEW did not have the same commitment to transfer grants to community boards as did OEO. There was a decided policy shift in the direction of allowing the current grantee to decide when the grant should be turned over to the community. In October 1973, the board held a workshop retreat. (This is not to be confused with the 1975 workshop retreat, described in the previous pages.)

At this workshop, Katz stated his view that the board at that time would have considerable difficulty in getting the grant. He went on to recommend that the board be reconstituted and that it should go through a substantial amount of training before Montefiore would ever trust the board with such monies. After this workshop, the bylaws were modified and a new board composition was developed. The membership was to consist of one third community people from the old board, one third professionals, and one third staff members. Although these proportions were never exactly observed, all three of these groups continued to be represented on the board during the period of 1975–76.

In addition to reviewing the history of the board, the weekend included a discussion of four models detailing proposed board functions developed by Katz and Smith (see appendix to this chapter). These models were submitted to a vote. The result indicated that most board members were in favor of full granteeship in the long run. In the short run, however, they favored a transition—taking place as described in models 2 or 3. Task forces were created for accomplishing these objectives.

The task forces were given mandates and assigned members and target dates. Among the assignments were the creation of new bylaws, detailed legal and financial options for an autonomous MLK, and design of training plans for board members.

PRESENT-DAY DEVELOPMENTS

Wait and See

The first event after the workshop was the resignation of one of the professional members because "he saw no hope." The reason he gave was that he felt that several community members were using the board as a political tool.

The task forces began to meet and work on their assignments. But after six months, this work ceased. However, a plan was developed to simulate granteeship with Katz as the board's overseer. This simulation of the board's real operation actually began in the fall of 1976. Since then, the composition of the board has changed to meet new HEW guidelines that prohibit staff membership on the board.

Who Needs a Board?

The law requires the existence of a board of trustees to be ultimately responsible for the "trust" over a nonprofit health center. The OEO neighborhood health centers created under Title II were to have "maximum feasible participation." As was noted in the previous chapter, there are multiple routes to community control. The external control route is best accomplished through some form of board. The problem is OEO ambivalence about such questions as who actually represents the community and, more importantly, who in these poverty communities is capable of handling responsibility over such grants. The solution has been to assemble an ambivalent mixed model to incorporate external control of the center. Real control was to be given to "trustees" of institutions such as Montefiore. There would be additional arrangements for an advisory board to represent the community.

In sum, the need for a board at MLK was externally created. It gave Wise and his activist professionals the legal legitimacy and access to funding sources they needed. In addition, their requirements for community access and acceptance were being accomplished through coopting procedures that were more far-reaching (such as training and employing hundreds of community residents) than the notion of merely establishing an advisory board. In reality, there was very little pressure for a board.

What Is the Community?

In the early planning days, it was obvious to Dr. Wise and his colleagues that the idea of defining just what comprised "the community" would not be easy in the South Bronx. This is consistent with the community power studies by Michael Aiken (1970) that show great variation in terms of how complex and pluralistic a community can be. Dispersion of power according to Aiken becomes greater in the following situations: location in the North, high degree of absentee ownership of real estate property, heterogeneous population, and lower socioeconomic status (p. 523). The South Bronx scores high on all four of these criteria. Therefore, the existence of a dispersed, pluralistic power structure in the South Bronx is not surprising.

Organizations faced with varying levels of uncertainty are driven to develop ways of reducing such uncertainty. The establishment of a functioning governing board at MLK would be a problem-producing task because of the pluralistic, dynamic political nature of the community. This heterogeneous makeup would actually increase uncertainty, requiring management to invest resources in dealing with the uncertainty.

In discussing why people run for boards in 1970, Wise provides a description of the self-serving interests typcially represented on boards in low-income areas (1970):

1.   To promote a particular health or health related cause like the cause of mentally retarded children.
2.   To influence the distribution of training positions, jobs in the center, the upgrading of certain staff, or the prevention of certain staff from being fired.
3.   To use the position of a board member as a means of getting a job in the health program.
4.   To control a major local institution . . . for increasing the power of a particular interest group.
5.   To protect the interest of health consumers.

In the Wise quote, we are provided a subtle glimpse of the MLK posture toward developing a community board. His negative stance developed into a clear strategy pursued by management and reflected in staff attitudes toward the board.

By 1974, the MLK staff's position via-a-vis the board began to coalesce. Table 5.2 presents the response to a survey administered in 1974 to 60 percent of the staff (234). The survey asked questions regarding how the staff viewed the advisory board, as well as about the possibility of the board taking over control of the HEW grant from Montefiore. The majority of staff were in favor of some sort of advisory board (62 percent). At the same time, the majority were opposed to the particular board as constituted taking over (60 percent). (Note, only 10 percent favored the board at that time.)

MLK BOARD STRATEGY

As was discussed in Chapter 3 on MLK strategy, there are both explicitly and consciously formulated strategies, as well as strategies that evolve in a subtle, nonexplicit manner, yet nonetheless represent strategies. The board strategy at MLK is consistent with Mintzberg's (1976a) view that "when a series of decisions related to some aspect of the organization exhibits some consistency over time, a strategy will be considered to have formed."

TABLE 5.2

MLK Staff Attitudes toward Community Advisory Board
(percent)

Does the possibility of the community advisory board taking
over the administration of the HEW grant from Montefiore . . .

. . . bothers me very much	54
. . . bothers me somewhat	20
. . . bothers me very little	9
. . . not a problem to me	13
	4.6 (no answer)
	100 (n = 234)

A. How likely do you feel that the present community advisory board will take
over administration of the HEW grant from Montefiore? Circle one number.

1. very likely	5
2. quite likely	4
3. somewhat likely	8
4. neutral–don't know	50
5. somewhat unlikely	9
6. quite unlikely	7
7. very unlikely	13
8. no answer	4
	100 (n = 234)

B. If the present community board were in charge of MLK's funds, how would
you feel?

1. strongly in favor	4
2. moderately in favor	3
3. slightly in favor	3
4. neither in favor nor opposed	26
5. slightly opposed	22
6. moderately opposed	29
7. strongly opposed	39
8. no answer	4
	100 (n = 234)

C. Do you feel the present advisory board is representative of the community?

1. yes, very representative	9
2. yes, somewhat representative	48
3. no, not representative	42
4. no answer	1
	100 (n = 234)

D. If there is a community advisory board, which of the following groups should have members on the board? (Select more than one.)

	Yes	No	Total
1. MLK staff	58	42	100 (n = 234)
2. MLK patients	62	38	100 (n = 234)
3. Local community leaders, not patients	38	62	100 (n = 234)
4. Local community members who are not patients	32	68	100 (n = 234)
	190		

E. Which of the following groups is *most* important to be represented on the board? (Select one.)

1. MLK staff	26
2. MLK patients	48
3. Local community leaders who are not patients	10
4. Local community members who are not patients	6
5. No answer	10
	100 (n = 234)

F. Are you in favor of having some sort of community advisory board?

1. strongly in favor	28
2. moderately in favor	21
3. slightly in favor	13
4. neither in favor nor opposed	27
5. slightly opposed	2
6. moderately opposed	1
7. strongly opposed	4
8. no answer	4
	100 (n = 234)

Source: Compiled by the author.

The strategy that developed was to delay, to cool it. Resources were invested in reducing the uncertainty implicit in the board's training and makeup. As late as fall 1976, the MLK director's viewpoint was to let the board function at a low energy level, to allow unfilled seats to remain vacant. By doing so she encouraged the cooling-it tendency. Achieving internal and external control was something for the future. Through 1976 the two strongest driving forces in that direction were HEW and Montefiore. This changed early in 1977 when MLK's director began more forcefully to develop a board.

The absence of a functioning board leaves MLK without the ongoing mechanism that Drucker (1973) calls for in all organizations: a review organ, a critical superior court to monitor top management; a mechanism to remove a top management that fails; and a strong public and community relations organ. As Drucker clearly indicates, organizations require boards to fulfill these three functions. From this book's standpoint, the scales that need balancing are currently in the following positions:

1. External versus internal community control. The balance is tilted almost totally toward the internal side. This tilt is made even more extreme by the outmigration to suburban areas of many of the "community" managers and workers. As a result, new mechanisms for community input and influence are clearly called for.

2. Local Bronx political agendas versus city, state, and federal political agendas. The infighting between Puerto Ricans and blacks in the Bronx (as partially played out on the earlier MLK board) has currently dissipated. The scale is now more balanced as it relates to MLK. Probably, little more than monitoring is needed at this point. Reasonable balance can be maintained through member selection on the emerging board.

3. Poverty class norms and behavior. The exercise of power and influence through particiation on boards is a "game" played by elite elements in society. Very clear, yet often implicit, rules of play have emerged for middle-class exercise of power on boards. For example, it is unacceptable for a middle-class board member to use his or her power to acquire a job for a family member or close friend at the institution on whose board he or she sits. However, it is more acceptable to use that power skillfully to get a job for a family member or friend at a neighboring or even competing institution. This is especially true of nonprofit institutions where board members are trustees.

   Poverty-class norms and behavior tend to be more direct in the use of power achieved through board membership. In the early years at MLK, board members sought direct favors from the organization, especially jobs for friends and family. This scale is now tilting toward the middle-class norms and behavior side. The selection and socialization of new board members will tend to encourage this pattern. This is beneficial to MLK because the funding sources play by middle-class norms and behavior.

4. Montefiore as paternalistic protector versus MLK independence. The January 1, 1978 deadline dictated by HEW will force coming to grips with the balancing of this scale. The solution will probably be to place some value on both sides of this scale. Through some special contractual arrangement, MLK could conceivably continue to benefit from Montefiore's protection and support. At the same time, the HEW mandate for independence could be fulfilled. This is the scale that currently absorbs the largest amount of attention. Its balance is the most precarious of all the scales both now and in the foreseeable future.

APPENDIX: POSSIBLE MLK BOARD RESPONSIBILITY MODELS*

In considering possible relationships of the board to the center, its administration, and Montefiore, we have, from time to time, discussed a variety of possible models. Recently, however, we concentrated on only the granteeship model to the exclusion of all others.

In its deliberations during the retreat it seems appropriate that the board again examine a variety of models to arrive, hopefully, at one which will both most usefully meet the needs of the center and those of the Board, both collectively and individually. Following is a brief description of four possible models. These are not by any means all the possible variations, but serve merely as a point from which to start the discussion.

1. *Full Granteeship*

The board is totally and legally responsible for the center, both collectively and individually.

All fiscal and policy decision, therefore, are board responsibility.

The center is independent and may have to carry its own labor contracts, hospital backup arrangements, malpractice insurance, fringe benefit program, and complete executive and administrative staff (i.e., purchasing, personnel, accounting, etc.) to carry out all phases of the activity.

2. *Granteeship and Contract Relationship*

The board is the grantee. However, it contracts for facilities administration with MHMC or any other institution.

Annually the board and the contractor agree in writing on the program for the coming year and the budget necessary to fulfill this program. The contractor is responsible for the implementation of the program within the agreed budget. If, as a result of unexpected cost increases or diminution of income the program cannot be fulfilled, the contractor and the board will agree on a change in program to meet the new circumstances. Failure to agree within (say) 30 days will allow the contractor to make necessary program adjustments to keep the center fiscally whole.

If the board, in the course of the contract year, wishes to change the program, such changes can be implemented by mutual agreement.

The total administration and personnel relations are the responsibility of the contractor under this arrangement.

3. *Mixed Model*

Montefiore is the grantee.

The Board has explicit consultation and approval authority specifically in:

a. hiring the project director and his/her immediate deputies

b. the program and budget

c. all other program and grant applications

The board has a complete committee structure and has policy input into ongoing center activities.

4. *Advisory Model*

MHMC is the grantee.

The board serves as an informational interface with the community, representing community interests to the center and vice versa.

The board consults with and advises administration on program decisions and assists administration in securing funds and presenting the community's point of view to third parties such as HEW.

---

*Memorandum from Mo Katz and Deloris Smith to MLK Board, November 1975.

A wise man once said that the best team is that team made up of one
person. There are no conflicts, frustrations, or uncertainty.

> Benjamin Siegel, "Organization of the Primary Care
> Team," *Pediatric Clinics of North America* 21, no. 2 (May
> 1974): 343.

TRADE-OFFS

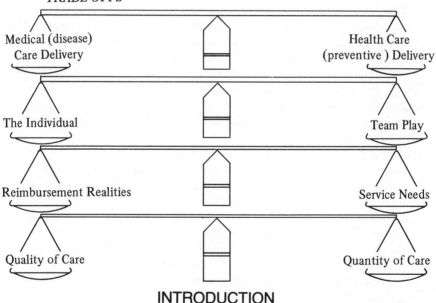

Medical (disease) Care Delivery — Health Care (preventive) Delivery

The Individual — Team Play

Reimbursement Realities — Service Needs

Quality of Care — Quantity of Care

INTRODUCTION

Herbert Simon (1967) provides a description that is also very fitting
for primary health care teams:

> Organizing a professional school or an R&D department is very
> much like mixing oil and water: it is easy to describe the intended

product, less easy to produce it. And the task is not finished when the goals have been achieved. Left to themselves, the oil and water will separate again. So also with the disciplines and professions. Organizing, in these situations, is not a once and for all activitity. It is a continuing administrative responsibility, vital for the sustained success of the enterprise (p.16).

The primary health care team as an ideal form of health care delivery is easy to describe and generally makes a great deal of sense. Nevertheless, it was the MLK experience that translating this ideal into reality can take over five years. And when the teams finally functioned effectively, the oil and water began to separate. Even though MLK is nationally known for its successful primary health care teams, there are problems and pressures that could eventually lead to the end of team care in this situation.

As noted in Chapters 1 and 2, MLK is noted for two important organizational design innovations: the primary health care team (Parker, 1972) and the use of a matrix type of organizational structure (Beckhard, 1972). The organizational model presented in Chapter 2 made reference to a component called sociotechnical arrangements. This component will be examined in this chapter as well as the next. This chapter focuses on the microsociotechnical design at MLK, namely, the primary health care teams. The next chapter will focus on the macrosociotechnical system, that is, the way in which teams are coordinated with each other and with other subunits of the organization.

The scales that require special managerial attention with regard to the function of teams are:

1. Medical (disease) care delivery versus health care (preventive) delivery. The U.S. health system has been increasingly criticized for focusing on illness and disease (Illich, 1974; Carlson, 1975; Mechanic, 1969; Kissick, 1970) rather than on helping to prevent people from becoming sick through education and preventive services. A comprehensive health center must provide both types of services and allocate its resources in both areas. The balancing issue revolves around how much of what kinds of services in the various levels of care should be provided. As shall be noted, this scale is closely related to how care is financed and what is considered to be a reimbursable service.

2. The individual prima donnas versus team players. The dominant figure in the U.S. health system is and will be for the foreseeable future the physician. He or she is trained to be autonomous, be the ultimate decider and be in charge of other health providers. The health care team is designed for collaboration among disciplines

without dominance by any one group. Therefore, unless the training of physicians and the legal and institutional infrastructures supporting physician dominance change, then the dilemma of having physicians be team players will continue to emerge. The managerial response at MLK has included selecting physicians with proclivity for team care as well as special training and development activities for the teams.

3. Reimbursement realities versus service needs. The delivery of health care in a poverty underserved area poses a severe health-financing dilemma, namely, balancing the service needs with what the third-party payers are willing to finance. For example, if home visits and help in getting lead-based paint off the walls of apartments are needed health services, the management must face the issue of finding a way to finance such a service, as Medicaid will not reimburse MLK for sending family health workers out into the homes.

4. Quality of care versus quantity of care. The dilemma in this area is how much to invest in seeing large numbers of patients versus how much to invest in ensuring the quality of their treatment. The conflict comes into play when management must decide how to use the time of the providers (how many hours auditing charts, and so on).

THE IMAGE OF A PRIMARY CARE TEAM

The task of providing comprehensive primary care is a great deal more uncertain than other types of personal health care. Table 6.1 contrasts elements of primary care with tertiary care. The contrasts indicate greater degrees of task uncertainty, as well as the need for more interdependence among different disciplines in a primary care setting. Note that primary care is concerned with the health of a specified population at risk, providing care for problems for which there are few therapeutic regimens, providing care of an interpersonal nature that is long term and where decisions are often intuitive.

Organization and management research (Burns and Stalker, 1961; Lawrence and Lorsch, 1967; Galbraith, 1973; Tushman and Nadler, 1976) indicate that the conditions of task uncertainty and high dependence surrounding primary care call for a sociotechnical arrangement characterized by decentralization, low formalization, peer leadership and decision making, fully interconnected communication, high capacity for feedback and error catching, and low dependence on a supervisor. Therefore the ideal primary health team has these design characteristics.

TABLE 6.1

Dichotomy of Health Care

Primary Care	Tertiary Care
Population at risk (under health pressure)	Individual in need
Health care (total sociophysical health care)	Medical care (diagnostic-therapeutic care)
Interpersonal	Technical (impersonal)
Generalist	Specialist
10 to 15 percent of all diagnoses explain complaints	80 to 90 percent of all diagnoses underlies indices of suspicion
Represent 90 percent of health care need	Represent 10 percent of medical need
Few therapeutic regimens	Extensive treatment protocols
Matrix organizations	Hierarchical
Placebo	Specific prescription
Office	Hospital
Home/community	Institutional environment
Probability theory	Reductionistic
Intuitive treatment	Deductive treatment
Long term patient population	Episodic patient population
Comprehensive treatment	Singular treatment
Data: interview	Diagnostic studies
Triage	Referral
Patient and physician are peers	Physician is dominant over patient

Note: Levels of care are defined as: tertiary—highly specialized, technologically based intensive care, centralized in large medical centers frequently located in universities; secondary—specialized consultant care that should be based in large-sized community hospitals; primary—treatment based in offices or health centers with a few "holding" or observation beds close to where people live and work (White, 1973).

Source: William Kissick and Samuel Martin, "Organization of Personal Health Services," in *Resource Book on Health and Behavioral Sciences in Health Administration*, ed. Kent Peterson (Washington, D.C.: Association of University Programs in Health Administration, 1977).

DEFINITION AND ROLE OF A PRIMARY HEALTH CARE TEAM

In order to establish a team, a clear notion is needed regarding the services the team is to provide. At MLK such a notion was provided early by its definition of family- and community-oriented comprehensive care.

This definition stated that services should range on a broad spectrum, from very specific acute problems to health problems caused by inadequate housing and nutritional problems. Although the original role concepts for the team were very general and vague, they provided sufficient guidelines for deciding upon the mix of disciplines necessary to delivery services. The team members found on the MLK primary health care team include the following:

Family health workers. Family health workers (five or six) are or were neighborhood residents trained as generalists in home nursing, health education, and social advocacy skills. They assist nurse practitioners and physicians in recording routine health and social histories, as well as undertaking medication checks. They place reports into the medical records covering the health and social problems affecting each family member and of the family as a whole. They provide home care, bedside nursing for homebound patients, supervision of healthy babies, diet and medication review, and posthospital follow-up. In their advocacy role, they help patients with housing, social welfare, and school-related problems. In their health educator's role, they investigate hazards in the home, the presence of lead paint, and so on.

Nurse practitioner. Nurse practitioners, one or two per team, provide three basic functions. First, they act as coordinators for many of the families, making certain that family care plans are developed, that appointments are made for routine care, and that family health records are reviewed. Second, they are responsible for supervising the work of several family health workers. Third, they perform duties in the care of healthy babies, normal pre- and postnatal care of mothers, routine adult preventive care, and some psychiatric crisis care.

Pediatrician. These physicians (one per team) are primarily responsible for acutely ill children. They also act as consultant and teacher to other members of the team.

Internist. Internists (one or two per team) are responsible for providing adult care to appointment and walk-in patients. They, too, have a consultant and teacher responsibility to other team members.

In addition to these members, primary health care teams have medical assistants who provide service to two teams. They prepare patients, assist during interviews (translate where necessary), assist during examinations, and carry out such procedures as blood pressure, specimen collection, urine testing, preparations for pap smears, and so on. Each unit has a receptionist and secretary as well as a unit manager.

The role of a team is clear, or at least so thought the MLK staff as they started the center. All that was necessary, they felt, was to put all these people together and they would then perform as a team. They did not realize, until after some trial-and-error experiences, that pouring oil and water into the same container, that is, mixing disciplines, does not complete the mix.

BACKGROUND OF PRIMARY CARE TEAMS AT MLK

It is not by accident that the primary health care team was able to develop so fully at MLK. The original proposal to OEO clearly contained the rudiments of the primary health care team as it exists today at MLK. The roots of the MLK primary health care team had their origin in the home-care program developed by Dr. Martin Cherkasky in the late 1940s (Cherkasky, 1949). The team, made up of internist, nurse, physical therapist, social worker, secretary, and driver, provided care for chronically ill people at home. Basically, the team operated like an in-hospital team. Later, Dr. George Silver developed a preventive treatment team that built on Cherkasky's team, broadening the service to include treatment and health maintenance care. Both Cherkasky and Silver had a strong commitment to innovation in primary care. It was Silver who directly influenced Wise in the proposal that eventually became the OEO-funded Dr. Martin Luther King, Jr. Health Care Center.

The original concept incorporated physicians, public health nurses, and community residents who gave outreach home and clinic care. This, in fact, is the pattern followed in the early days of MLK.

THE PROBLEMS OF TEAM CARE
IN THE EARLY DAYS

As noted above, the health team consisted of pediatricians, internists, public health nurses, and family health workers. However, it was soon discovered that the act of merely placing different professionals on a team with the intention of providing comprehensive team care often resulted in fragmented and inconsistent care.

The first few years of teams at MLK were filled with problems—and for good reason. There was no clearly articulated view of what a health care team should do. No specific health care delivery goals existed. The roles of the various members on the team were not clear. It was hard to differentiate clearly what the job function of a family health worker was, in contrast to the function of a public health nurse. Also, the overlap between public health nurses and physicians often became blurred. The information systems, including the medical record system, were not structured in a way in which they could facilitate team care delivery. Most important was the fact that specific team processes for communicating and making decisions had not been developed yet. An outcome was that the first three years of the center's operation provided the development of a number of innovative responses to these difficulties.

Team development during the first few years was carried out by trial and error. It was possible for MLK to develop teams in this experimental way in the early days without resulting in total chaos, as there were ample resources in the organization. The reason was that the project was well funded, without an overwhelming patient load. By 1970, years after the center's founding, some of the problems in delivering team-oriented care had been overcome.

A major improvement came about as a result of the use of the problem-oriented medical record as developed by Dr. Weed. The MLK health center is noted for its successful integration of the problem-oriented medical record into team care (see Appendix C for details of the problem-oriented medical record system at MLK).

The teams might have continued to function and improve themselves by trial and error if it hadn't been for a major developmental milestone in MLK's history. The rapid expansion from the small Bathgate Avenue Center to the large Third Avenue Center almost overnight moved MLK from a two-team system to an eight-team system. Once this growth took place, it was no longer possible to patch up problems informally. This created a major organizational crisis. At the same time, stresses on the teams were also being reflected as stresses at the managerial and organizational levels. These managerial problems and the events surrounding them will be discussed in more detail in the next chapter.

The team development work of the MIT group is responsible for the next phase in the progress of the primary health care teams at MLK.

TEAM DEVELOPMENT INTERVENTION— ACTION RESEARCH

The work of the MIT group grew directly out of the organization development orientation in vogue at that time in many industrial and business organizations (Beckhard, 1969; Hornstein et al, 1971). The thrust of the MIT organization development efforts can be called the action research mode of intervention. "Action research" is a term coined by

Kurt Lewin (1948) that refers to the orderly collection of data on real social or organizational problems that are systematically fed back to the people experiencing the problem in order to facilitate and provide a basis for their problem solving. The data collection and feedback occur on an ongoing basis so that organizational members can make changes, evaluate the outcome of those changes, and then make new changes. This occurs either when the first solution did not work or to maximize the success of the first intervention.

The crucial feature of the action research mode is that the consultant, generally an outside behavioral science consultant, acts as a facilitator to enable the team to solve its own problems, not as an expet to tell it just what to do (Argyris, 1970).

The MIT group began work with several teams by systematically collecting information regarding how the teams were functioning as well as identifying some of their current problems. Guiding the data collection and the work of the MIT group was a very specific orientation to teams and team development. In addition to being committed to an action research mode of working with teams, the MIT group had a set of basic assumptions about the benchmarks of an effective team. These assumptions included (Fry, Lech, and Rubin, 1974):

1. A work group is not defined as a team unless its members are actually interdependent in order to accomplish a task.
2. Teams need to establish explicit and shared goals that constitute their working contract with each other.
3. Team members collaboratively arrive at role descriptions, based directly upon the explicit goals and objectives of the team.
4. Once the goals and roles are established, the team must develop processes for communication, problem solving, decision making, and conflict management.
5. The team must develop the ability to deal with interpersonal and personal issues and dilemmas brought about by interaction in the work setting.

Figure 6.1 provides a summary of the MIT group's basic orientation to team development. This orientation has been further developed and refined by this group and is presented in a workbook (Rubin et al., 1975). The MIT group began working with each of the teams involved in this developmental activity by feeding back the results of a questionnaire.

Results of the interviews and questionnaires indicated that there was unnecessary duplication of effort, things did not always get done, meetings were ineffective, team members were unclear about their roles, teams had no clear objectives, and communication was sloppy—all leading to frustration. Based on the teams' reaction to the data, the MIT

FIGURE 6.1

Team Development

Objective: To impart knowledge and behavioral skills to members so they can more effectively manage and issues outlined below.

Team Development Process:

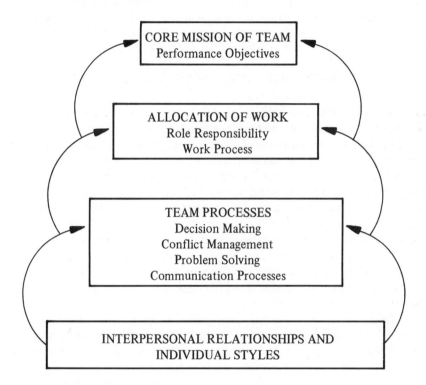

Initially a team consultant works with a team in carrying out the processes. However, the consultant, in collaboration with the team, works to institutionalize and build in the capacity for the team to carry through on the process without reliance on a consultant. In order for this to occur, normative and structural changes must occur. Normatively, the team needs to develop a culture that explicitly supports the use of social interventions to regulate team processes, especially those related to decision-making communication, allocation of work, and planning. Structurally this is facilitated by formally allocating team time and resources to diagnosis and planning improvement strategies.

Source: Compiled by the author.

group began working on team goals, roles, and processes as outlined above. The team development work was carried out over a one-year period. Typically, each team took part in about 12 half-day meetings during this time.

The results of the team development work with the MIT group were very positive. It should be pointed out, however, that an extremely important organizational change was taking place simultaneously that made it possible for the team development work to be successful, namely, the implementation of the matrix structure discussed in Chapter 7.

THE OIL AND WATER BEGIN TO PART

In 1977, MLK is still a model for primary health care teams. However, there are clear indications that Simon's (1967) prophecy of the oil and water separation problem is coming true at MLK. First, team members often complain about their work in ways they hadn't before. For example, nurses and family health workers now object to the fact that physicians "are not interested in a collaborative team approach to health care." Team members often fail to attend team meetings, which were originally an important occasion for conferencing about client families and coordinating team activities. At times such meetings are called off. New sets of professional cleavages are beginning to form, especially between nurses and pediatricians. Finally, there is less of an overall sense of taking part in something creative and new. Work on the teams is becoming just another job for many.

There are several reasons for the deterioration in the primary health care teams at MLK. The Simon analogy of the natural tendency for oil and water to separate is in part an explanation of what is happening at MLK. As Simon points out, such a mix is not a one-time process; once oil and water are combined, it needs to be continuously stirred. Once interdisciplinary primary health care teams are developed, it is undoubtedly necessary to "stir them" to provide some kind of continual process to ensure that they stay together and work collaboratively. There has been very little team development activity since the MIT group began its work with the teams. Several teams have tried to initiate their own team development activities. Most of these activities have faltered after several weeks. The lack of continued attention to keeping the teams together makes this cohesion difficult. This is particularly the case when team members have left and been replaced by others who never took part in the original team development activities. This is only one cause and may, in fact, not be the major cause of the deterioration of the health care teams at MLK.

The second, and perhaps more serious, force working against the primary health care team notion is the direct result of external financial pressures placed on MLK. MLK's resources are becoming tighter and tighter. With the lessening of resources, increased pressure is placed on teams and individual team members to become more cost-effective.

The conventional wisdom assumes that the health team as developed at MLK is a more expensive model of delivering health care than traditional physician and institutional modes of primary health care. In fact, overall, it is—in part because the health team is providing a broader spectrum of services than most alternative forms of primary health care. The criteria for evaluating cost-effectiveness must take this into account. When not accounted for, the result is that MLK teams are evaluated on the basis of traditional health outcomes (number of patients seen for acute and chronic care by physicians) in spite of the fact that much of their energy and resources are funneled into such activities as health education, preventive medicine, and public health activities, all carried out by a variety of health providers.

These unwarranted comparisons of apples and oranges continue to be made, resulting in such conclusions as reported in the New York Times: "The Dr. Martin Luther King Health Center in the Bronx spends $75 per patient visit, far more than it would cost to treat a person in a doctor's office" (September 13, 1971, pp. 1, 38). When more careful research has been conducted, the evidence demonstrated that, comparing costs of providing specific units of services at OEO neighborhood health centers, including MLK, versus alternative institutional providers, the health centers were competitive (Sparer and Anderson, 1972).

Another problem affecting cost-effectiveness is what third-party payers, such as Medicaid, are willing to reimburse. How do you compensate a unique group of health workers, able to provide services normally supplied by professionals one rung up the ladder, for instance, nurse practitioners, especially in the pediatrics area, who perform many of the services normally provided by the pediatrician? This has created a serious reimbursement problem. In earlier days, it was creatively circumvented by MLK but currently it is increasingly becoming an issue. For example, as competition for pediatric patients increases, some pediatricians will not authorize reimbursement for work done by nurse practitioners.

The equilibrium of the primary care team has been upset at MLK largely due to increased environmental uncertainty. There are indications that this source of uncertainty will continue to prevail at MLK and hence affect the overall team concept. Therefore a need exists to readjust the team structure and its organizational processes. New trade-offs will have to be made and the scales will have to be rebalanced.

IMPLICATIONS OF THE TEAM CONCEPT

Benjamin Siegel (1974), in a review of the primary care team literature, indicated that many different kinds of team models were then operative, and that there was controversy over the proper "mix" of who should be on a team. Alternative structures that he found were physician, nurse, community health worker (family health worker); physician, nurse, community health worker, social worker; physician and nurse; nurse and health workers; physician, nurse, community health worker, mental health worker; family health advocate, family health associate with physician in a consulting role; physician, social worker, physical therapist, team secretary, automobile driver; and physician and social worker.

The only conclusion Siegel could draw at the time was that teams provided the best delivery mode for primary care, and that composition depended on a variety of factors. In other words, the mix was not easily predetermined. Such a conclusion at that time encouraged a growing number of primary care team advocates, most of whom received their "religion" from MLK, to attempt to disseminate the MLK approach.

The work of Siegel (1974) and Parker (1972), as well as that performed at the Institute for Health Team Development at Montefiore, plus teams created by the Student American Medical Association, were all influenced by the MLK experience. However, a short few years later we not only must return to questions raised by Siegel about the proper mix of professionals. We also are faced with deeper questions about whether teams make any sense at all. As noted in this chapter, oil and water seem to be separating at MLK. This is underway before other places have even started the initial mix.

It is necessary to examine what this means for the primary health team at MLK as a model. First, it was demonstrated in this chapter that the task uncertainty and interdependence needs in a primary care setting do appear to call for an organic team type of delivery structure as developed at MLK. There has, as stated before, been tightening of resources since the early 1970s when the MLK teams were developed into their current configuration. The primary organizational reaction to these shifts has been pressure for seeing more patients.

This state of affairs tends to validate such criticisms as those raised early in the OEO neighborhood health center movement about the cost-effectiveness of this type of care, which contend that MLK team care is more costly than traditional modes of care. On the surface the criticism cannot be refuted; it costs more to run MLK on a per-patient basis than it does more traditional ambulatory care facilities serving the same number of patients. As previously indicated, this is deceptive because it has not been determined whether this is due to the fact that the same services cost more or whether the primary care teams at MLK are offering different, more costly services—such as those associated with prevention and education that are generally nonreimbursable and hence get figured into the costs of reimbursable services (albeit hidden costs). If this is the case, then the problem is not that primary care teams are more costly, but that rather they are offering noncomparable services.

Another alternative is that health teams are indeed more expensive for the same services. The truth is probably some of both. MLK has not yet resolved the issue. In part, this is because of the continued availability of federal grant money to pick up deficits.

Today, however, management must come to grips with the conflict between what government is disposed to pay for and what MLK perceives as good comprehensive care. The response has been to primarily stress quantity instead of quality. The internal control system monitors and pushes for more patients per practitioner as the population base dwindles. This has resulted in internal competition for patients.

A PROPOSED RESPONSE

The dilemma is no longer how to supply family-oriented care but how to become cost-effective. This as yet has not been faced. Action should probably occur first on an organizationwide basis, with adjustments to be made in the structure and functioning of the primary health care team. The strategic planning prescribed in Chapter 9 is the first step in this process.

In searching for solutions to cost-effectiveness, it will be necessary to reexamine the internal structure of the team and the allocation of team resources. Figure 6.2 adds some new parameters to the design of the primary health care team. Rather than visualizing a team as having one structure and one set of operating principles, it may be more accurate, and ultimately lead to a better use of resources in a cost-effective manner, to differentiate more carefully the type of work carried out by such an interdisciplinary team.

Figure 6.2 includes multiple dimensions. First, there are options of care, ranging from individual to community care. Second, there is the target of care ranging from acute medical intervention to preventive psychosocial activity. Running parallel to the target is a dimension indicating the depth of the intervention.

FIGURE 6.2

Organization of Work on a Primary Health Care Team

Focus of Care

Depth of Intervention	Target	Individual	Couple	Family	Community
Less	Acute Medical				
	Chronic Medical				
	Preventive Medical				
	Acute Psychosocial				
	Chronic Psychosocial				
More (low accessability, high individuality	Preventive Psychosocial				

Source: Compiled by the author.

Each cell of this matrix can be examined to help guide decisions regarding how an individual team should be structured around each type of task.* For example, the protocols for individual acute and chronic care

---

*Table 6.2 presents a framework for analyzing the degree of task interdependence between different types of providers on health teams at MLK (Smith and Martin, 1973).

require very little team interaction and collaboration, whereas preventive medicine would have to draw on a more collaborative approach. The point of such an examination would be to evaluate what is the appropriate configuration for the variable demands of the task. The result will undoubtedly lead to multiple monitors and a more effective utilization of manpower with clearer accountability control.

RECOMMENDED ORGANIZATION DESIGN ADJUSTMENTS

The proposal for addressing team problems at MLK requires the following organization and managerial design adjustments:

1. Medical (disease-oriented) care versus health (preventive-oriented) care delivery. Currently, the balance is tipping in the direction of medical care delivery. Balancing in this area would involve obvious trade-offs between financial considerations represented by the utilization of time and staff for nonreimbursable activities and the value position about health and the actual community health and service needs. Balancing will require a careful analysis of the service and provider requirements in the matrix in Figure 6.2.
2. The individual prima donnas versus team play. It has been mentioned that oil and water are separating. As they separate, individualistic team members, especially physicians, become less interested in collaborative team play. The balance is definitely swinging away from team play and heading toward the reemergence of the solo prima donnas. As will be noted in the chapter on organizational processes, there is probably a need for this solo work in certain areas involving routine and programmable decisions. A model for deciding under what conditions team play is called for and when individualistic play is desirable is presented in Chapter 8.
3. Reimbursement realities versus service requirements. The external financing system has clearly telegraphed the message that health care costs are too high and that reimbursement will eventually be limited to certain basic services. It is a fact that in the MLK patient population, many nonreinbursable services have a greater potential for exerting favorable impact on the health status of patients than do reimbursable services. Yet, if the organization is to survive, the scale must tilt toward having to be responsive to reimbursement realities. The balancing of this scale will only be possible if the organization can expand its patient base and generate more revenues to cover nonreimbursable, yet needed services, such as home visits and

TABLE 6.2

Functions Carried Out That Affect Other Team Members

	Family Health Worker (FHW)	Public Health Nurse (PHN)	Pediatrician (Ped)	Internist (Int)
Family Health Worker		1. Requests reasonable and doc. requests for information 2. Assists with problem patients and home visits. 3. Family unit social problems 4. Family unit no-shows	1. Requests reason and doc. requests for information 2. Assists with problem 3. Chronic care 4. Family unit social problems	1. Requests reasonable and doc. requests for information. 2. Assists with problems— good notes 3. Full intake done
Public Health Nurse	1. Postpartum visits 2. Provides good family and MD information on problem patients 3. Family unit regular no-shows 4. Appoints patients behind health maintenance	1. Provides coverage for other FHWs 2. Assists in problem cases 3. Covers home visits during vacation	1. Provides coverage for others' patients 2. Assists with problems 3. Walk-ins seen 4. Referral to each other 5. Ratio of scheduled appointments to other PHN	1. Refers well child and babies for nurse-practitioner 2. Teaches and supervises 3. Health maintenance reviews and status	1. Refers pre-natals and well adults for care 2. Chronic problem care referred 3. Teaches—notes 4. Number of Paps done

Pediatrician	1. Completes health maintence work-ups before appointment 2. Referral for family unit 3. Home visit request 4. Postpartum referral 5. Family units and resolves complicated problems	1. Sees well children and routine problems 2. Family unit and resolves complex problems 3. Health maintenance referrals	1. Cross coverage Walk-in coverage	1. Refers patients to pediatrician in need of care with note
Internist	1. Completes health maintenance work-ups before appointment 2. Referral for family unit 3. Home visit request 4. Family unit regular and social problems	1. Sees well adults 2. Family unit and resolves complex problems 3. Handles chronic care problems 4. Family unit for family planning	1. Refers patients to internist in need of care with note	1. Cross covers and keeps notes patient-oriented as to maximize continuity.

Source: Deloris Smith and Edward Martin, "Evaluation of Quality of Medical Care Delivery by Ambulatory Health Care Teams," unpublished paper, 1973.

preventive care. This also means that the existing center staff will have to increase productivity rates, treating more patients with the same resources, while holding costs constant.

4. Quality of care versus quantity of care. Consistent with the tilt of the other team scales, this one is being pushed toward quantity. There is a strong tradition at MLK that exerts considerable pressure on the organization for quality care, yet the early 1977 movement is clearly toward quantity. The scale is slightly tipped in favor of quantity and may continue more so if left untended. The trade-offs in this area are similar to the ones in the other scales: finance versus values. Readjustment calls for a new mix of service and appropriate adjustments in who the providers should be for each of the health teams.

7

ORGANIZATION DESIGN:
MACROSTRUCTURE

The systems structure (matrix) will never be the preferred form of organization; it is fiendishly difficult. But it is an important structure, and one that the organization designer needs to know and needs to understand—if only to know that it should not be used where other, simpler and easier structures will do the job (Drucker, 1973, p. 598).

TRADE-OFFS

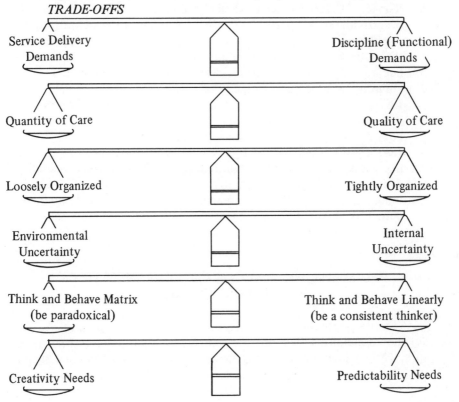

Service Delivery Demands	Discipline (Functional) Demands
Quantity of Care	Quality of Care
Loosely Organized	Tightly Organized
Environmental Uncertainty	Internal Uncertainty
Think and Behave Matrix (be paradoxical)	Think and Behave Linearly (be a consistent thinker)
Creativity Needs	Predictability Needs

INTRODUCTION

The previous chapter discussed the design of the health teams, the subunit organizations of MLK. This chapter focuses on the macrosociotechnical arrangements, the context within which these teams operate. In order to aid this analysis, a framework viewing both sociotechnical arrangements and organizational processes at MLK is presented.

The comprehensive interdisciplinary primary care, with an organization that frustrated such efforts, is documented, as is the transition to a new MLK design (largely with the help of Richard Beckhard). The new matrix structure was implemented in the early 1970s and successfully met the demands of the organization at that time. By 1975, the demands changed and as a result placed new strains on design and managers. These strains were still creating problems early in 1977. In order to deal with these strains, the following trade-offs need managing:

1. Service delivery demands versus discipline demands. The question of providing an appropriate mix of services to a defined patient population based on market information versus providing services that different disciplines—pediatrics, internal medicine, and so on— decide is appropriate regardless of market considerations.
2. Quantity of care versus quality of care.
3. Environmental uncertainty versus internal uncertainty. Determining the proper mix of capacity to handle uncertainty from the environment versus uncertainty generated internally.
4. Loosely organized versus tightly organized. Existence of discretion and slack resources versus tightly controlled and no slack resources.
5. Thinking and behaving matrix versus thinking and behaving unidimensionally. Actively managing paradoxical and conflicting demands versus dealing sequentially with conflicting demands, thus not bringing conflict out into the open.

FRAMEWORK: LEVELS OF ORGANIZATIONAL FUNCTIONING

The sociotechnical arrangements at MLK, as well as the organizational processes, provide vehicles for managing the above trade-offs. The sociotechnical arrangements at MLK discussed in this chapter and the organizational processes discussed in the following chapter are analyzed according to how they contribute to accomplishing four organizational functions or operations defined below.

The framework divides organizational functioning into four levels of operation.* The first level is steady state operation, that is, the ongoing regular routines of the organization. The organization operates and spends a certain percentage of its time doing such operations as routinely seeing patients, filling prescriptions, doing labwork and x-rays, attending regular committee meetings, filling out reports, reading reports, reviewing the work of others, and monitoring the budget.

Unfortunately, all organizations break down and require repair operations. Organizations function at this second level only part of the time and must frequently deal with crises of varying magnitude. These range from responding to an unexpected rate of absenteeism one day to conflict among departments, budget crises, or union problems. Most organizations introduce certain new innovative operations (the third category).

The fourth category is self-renewal operations, which refers to activities, time, and resources invested in diagnosing and developing ways of improving the first three levels of operations. Self-renewal is the major factor in determining the long-term health of an organization and is characterized by a negative entropy process in which extra energy is stored and conserved (Katz and Kahn, 1966).

An organization's sociotechnical arrangements and its managerial processes should facilitate all four levels. Organizations vary in the degree of how much time they should devote to each level. The key factor determining the importance of each of the four levels is the amount of uncertainty the organization faces. The greater the uncertainty, the more organizational resources need to go to innovation and self-renewal (Lawrence and Lorsch, 1967).

Table 7.1 presents a summary of how the four levels of operation would apply to MLK, and shows how each level requires different design and process characteristics to be effective. Thus, it provides an evaluation of the current status of sociotechnical and organizational processes at MLK. The table also summarizes the implications of this analysis for MLK. These will be discussed later in this and the next chapter.

The central points that need to be underscored from the material in Table 7.1 before examining the development of MLK's matrix design are:

---

*The four levels of organization functioning were first introduced to the author by Dr. Kenneth Pollock, who attributes the formulation to Dr. Matthew Miles.

TABLE 7.1

Levels of Organizational Functioning: Design Implications for MLK

Levels of Function	Conditions for Effectiveness	Current Assessment of MLK	Implications
Steady state operation: ongoing regular routines of the organization, predictable, programmable, low uncertainty, low information processing requirements.	Rational systems design—patient flow, protocols, management information system, standard operating procedures.	Excellent patient information system: Patient flow, protocols, and routine care procedures well designed. Management information system limited to catching quality errors and monitoring productivity. Teams need to be restructured. Matrix design not functioning, well out of balance. Support services functioning well.	Properly implemented and managed matrix. Develop new management information system (both sides of matrix).
Repair operation: non-routine problems, search for solution often unanalyzable, time pressures, often conflict, parties, and priorities.	Information search capacity, flexible problem-solving capability, conflict management structures and processes, contingency plans.	Conflict and problems worked on at team level need restructuring: Conflicts between quantity and quality go unmanaged. Matrix management that should facilitate explicit conflict and bargaining not occurring. Control systems geared toward avoiding error rather than error-embracing (learning from mistakes).	Reinforce matrix structure for guiding problem solving. Encourage open conflict management. Develop error-embracing control systems.

Innovative operation: Organizationally new and novel approaches to the task, management and organizational design generally imported from the environment (new knowledge, new developments from other organizations).	Environmental-scanning capability, appropriate boundary-spanning network, to keep up to date. Managerial and organizational capacity to evaluate, decide on, and implement innovations. Existence of some slack resources generally needed.	No structure for systematically linking organization to relevant domains (medical, political, financial). No structure of processes for facilitating the development of new innovations in service or organizational areas.	Develop boundary-spanning networks to monitor innovations. Set up top group for strategic planning organization design, and human resource management.
Self-renewal operation: Investing time and resources in diagnosing and developing improved ways of carrying out steady state, repair, and innovative operation.	Value commitment to self-diagnosis and improvement (preventive medicine, orientation to organize functioning), capacity for diagnosing managerial and organizational systems and organizational change capability.	Little proactive activity in last ten years. Strategy formation largely reactive, incrementalism. Moderately high value commitment to self-renewal, yet no significant resource commitment.	Set aside resources and time for self-renewal. Reward lower level self-renewal activities.

Source: Compiled by the author.

1. That each level of organizational functioning requires different structural and process mechanisms for effective operation.
2. Steady state operation makes the most use of rational managerial and organizational design procedures that enable the organization to arrange itself in such a manner as to perform tasks in a maximally predictable and controlled way. Thus the tools most useful in this area are management science work-flow design techniques, budget and control system design, and standing plans.
3. Repair operation requires organizational structures and processes that provide the capacity to handle conflict and to engage in nonprogrammed decision making. The crucial factor in repair operations is the ability to respond flexibly and with minimal time lag.
4. Innovative operations require structures and processes for monitoring the environment for innovations as well as mechanisms for putting innovations on stream. The organization must also possess risk capital or slack resources to engage in innovative operation. At MLK, for example, physicians need education time to keep up with new innovations. The organization must be in the position to provide in-service training to the end that new learning can be transferred to other organization members. The same processes are required on the management side in the categories of management development and new managerial practices.
5. Self-renewal operation is based above all on a normative commitment on the part of management regarding the virtue of taking time out to improve organizational functioning at the three other levels. This needs to be accompanied by specific structural and resource commitments devoted to ascertain that the self-renewal mode becomes institutionalized. Some organizations engage in annual top management strategic planning activities, others in regular self-diagnosis. (MLK's commitment to workshops is an example of a self-renewal activity.)

THE DEVELOPMENT OF THE MLK MATRIX STRUCTURE

Harold Wise and his early colleagues at MLK had teams in mind from the start. George Silver was his senior mentor and had advocated and developed primary teams in the past, specifically the family home care team. As indicated in the last chapter, no attention was paid to how to design an organizational structure that supported and encouraged team delivery.

This lack of an organizational structure resulted in a great deal of confusion and at times frustration. Initially, the problems could be overcome, however, because the organization was small enough to rely on informal corrective actions to compensate for an inadequate organizational structure. Under the recently introduced terms, MLK's steady state operation was poor, yet through informal interaction and the dedication to make things work, the repair operation took over much of what should have been steady state. Wise was able to use his charisma to mobilize individuals to work out problems caused by an inadequate organizational design.

The culture of MLK was one of experimentation and self-criticism. Hence, informal corrective mechanisms could function. However, this circumstance only prevailed until the opening of the Third Avenue Center, at which time MLK multiplied in size fourfold within a matter of months. The problem of poor organizational design became acute. Wise described the problem to Beckhard in the following terms (Wise et al., 1974, p. 70):

1. Health care is delivered to the families in the community through health teams composed of physicians, nurses and community based and center trained family health workers. We are having a lot of difficulties *in the operation of the health teams.*
2. We have problems with *the role of the public health nurse* on the teams. She is assigned as the coordinator and leader of the health team but this is a very strange role for her.
3. We have a lot of *communication difficulties* between the community oriented family health workers and the professionally trained physicians and nurses.
4. We have a number of problems in the area of *supervision*, particularly with first line supervisors who are mostly local residents whom we have trained.
5. We're having a lot of difficulty around *information flow* and *record keeping.* Patient records are often incomplete and in the wrong place at the wrong time. A number of referrals get lost between departments and between the center and the hospital.
6. Another problem for us is that the *overall management team* doesn't function very much as a team. Each functional department head, such as pediatrics or obstetrics, has his functional counterparts on the delivery team reporting to him and tends, naturally, to be more concerned with his own functional area than with the overall management of the center. This makes it difficult to get optimal decisions for the whole organization.
7. We're pretty sure that we're not properly organized *structurally* to manage this operation, but we don't know exactly how we should change our organization. [Emphasis added]

Dr. Wise was right. The organization design was working at cross-purposes to the intended team-care concept. Furthermore, management did not know how to improve on it. Management was clear on one thing: the type of service it wanted to provide for patients. It wanted the capability to evaluate health problems, diagnose disease causes, treat medical problems, diagnose and evaluate social and economic problems, treat social problems by legal and/or social action, and maintain a family's condition, once improved.

In order even to begin to provide such an array of services, it was clear that multiple disciplines were required. The problem as indicated in the last chapter was that task uncertainty was high. This brought a requirement for a subunit organization that was highly interdependent and problem-solving oriented, in other words, organically structured (Burns and Stalker, 1961; Galbraith, 1973). All team members possessed needed information for solving some but not all of their problems. Thus, sharing and collaboration were essential.

EVOLUTION OF THE SUBUNIT STRUCTURE

Figure 7.1 summarizes the core issues involved in various alternative organization designs. The amount of decision-making influence is the key trade-off. At the top left of the figure the discipline groups have total control. This is very much the case in traditional hospital departments where the authority structure is functionally or discipline oriented as is the reporting. The other end of the table represents a totally service-dominated structure where the authority is given over to a service structure as would exist with self-contained autonomous teams. There we see a variety of mechanisms for altering the balance between the two ends. For example, setting up special task forces can partially counterbalance the influence of either service or discipline orientation. The matrix represents equal influence for both disciplines and services. The result is a dual authority and dual reporting system.

The MLK structure was initially modeled from the traditional hospital structure in which the medical, nursing, and service disciplines each reported up its own hierarchy (the left side of the chart in Figure 7.1). Thus coordination between disciplines at the level of health care delivery was difficult. The reason was that each service had its own self-interest, which tended to pull them apart.

An alternative to the hospital's functionally dominated design would have been to shift all reporting and control to the team level, that is, to have self-contained team subunits, each with its own leader, responsible for all disciplines on the team. Thus, physicians, nurses, and family health

FIGURE 7.1

Alternative Organization Designs

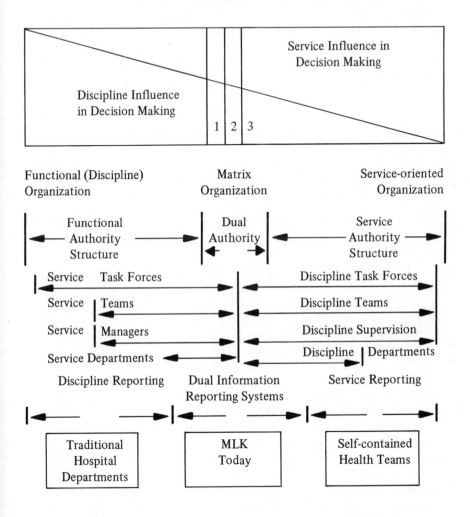

Source: Adapted from Jay Galbraith, *Designing Complex Organizations* (Reading, Mass.: Addison-Wesley, 1973), p. 114.

workers, as well as other personnel, would report to a supervisor common to all.

This alternative would have improved coordination at the cost of losing coordination and control within discipline groups. That is, nurses on one team would have no professional contact with nurses on another; there would be no overall professional supervisor for any of the disciplines. Each subunit would function much like a separate private clinic. Such a state of affairs could conceivably lead to lower levels of quality within disciplines and the lack of a colleague support system. By this is meant a system designed to help individuals within a discipline develop new and improved skills.

THE SOLUTION: THE MATRIX

A solution to the discipline (functional) versus service trade-off is to design an organization that stresses both and hence is built explicitly on competing demands. Because MLK is committed to fulfilling both discipline and service needs, an organization with a built-in, dual authority system is the preferred design. This is the matrix design. But promulgating a design with dual authority makes the matrix design fiendishly difficult to administer.

Figure 7.2 shows a matrix chart for MLK. The capabilities— pediatrics, internal medicine, nursing, and family health care—are assigned to a team in order to provide a specific mix of services. Team members report to their discipline chief for professional support, professional development, and issues of professional standards. In addition, each team member reports to a unit manager for administrative purposes, such as scheduling, budgeting, personnel matters, and relationship to other areas of the organization. Each unit manager is in charge of administering two teams. Both professional supervision and unit managers report to the director of health services.

The matrix design was implemented at MLK while at the same time Irwin Rubin's MIT group carried on team development consulting with individual teams. The matrix functioned quite well at MLK after its implementation. The teams were resocialized through the team development activities to relate and operate in new ways. The new organization structure fostered the continuation of these new operational patterns. The matrix design provided MLK with the integrating device needed to provide a complex service.

In this manner the scales were balanced from 1972 to 1974. Service versus discipline demands were equalized. There was an optimum mix of quantity and quality of care. The organization design had been modified from a dysfunctionally loose structure to one sufficiently tight to improve technical efficiency. Both environmental and internal

FIGURE 7.2

The Matrix Structure

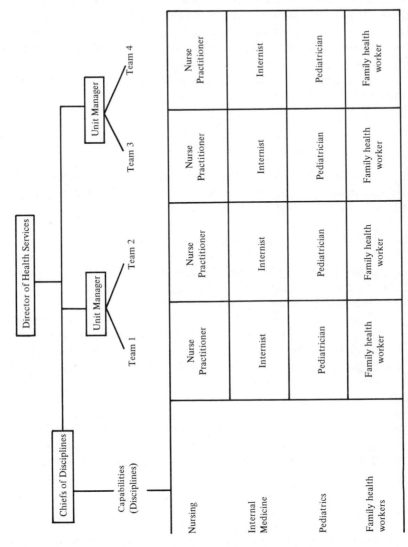

Source: From Richard Beckhard, "Organizational Implications of Team Building," in *Making Health Teams Work*, Richard Beckhard, Harold Wise, Irwin Rubin, and Aileen L. Kyte, eds. (Cambridge, Mass.: Ballinger, 1974), p. 78.

uncertainty were under control. The director of health services, Dr. Edward Martin, was "thinking and behaving matrix." At that time he was the key to the successful management of the matrix system. His medical background, coupled with a managerial orientation, enabled him to balance competing discipline demands and service demands. He was able to negotiate both sides of the matrix and recognize the importance of both.

THE MATRIX BEGINS TO DECOMPOSE

As observed in the last chapter, the teams in 1977 have been slowly coming apart. Harold Wise's quote of 1970 can be updated in 1977 to identify the following symptoms:

1. There are problems with the nurse practitioner's role.
2. There are beginnings of new communication difficulties between the family health workers and the professionally trained physicians.
3. The top team doesn't function much as a team.
4. Unit managers are not very effective.
5. There seems to be a drift toward stronger discipline orientation rather than team orientation. The drift is not improving services so much as defending vested discipline interests. The physicians are exploring the possibility of becoming a bargaining unit over issues of pay and job security.

Maybe Drucker was right after all. The matrix may be so fiendishly difficult to manage that the design self-destructs. Stanley Davis (1976) provides a glimpse at why the decomposition may be occurring at MLK. He identifies a set of conditions that are necesary for matrix designs to work:

1. The opportunities lost and difficulties experienced by favoring either a service or functional unity of command cannot be ignored.
2. There is a need for enriched information processing capacity because of uncertain and interdependent tasks.
3. Information planning and control systems operate along different dimensions of the structure simultaneously.
4. As much attention is paid to managerial behavior as to the structures. The organizational culture must actively support and believe in negotiated management. They have to "think matrix."

In addressing these organization design problems, it will be necessary for management to contend with balancing the following trade-offs: environmental uncertainty versus internal uncertainty, quantity of service versus quality of service, individual needs versus team needs, needs for autonomy versus needs for control, creativity needs versus predictability needs, and thinking matrix versus thinking unidimensionally.

Two factors can largely account for managerial and organizational problems with the matrix structure at MLK: (1) The level of environmental uncertainty has gone up. This is reflected in pressure for greater cost-effectiveness. Hence, quantity of care has increased, upsetting several internal balances. (2) The think matrix scale was thrown off balance when Edward Martin left MLK in January 1974. His unique combination of professional medical background, coupled with a sophisticated managerial orientation, enabled him to see and understand the trade-offs and paradoxes built into the matrix structure. He was also capable of personally managing both sides of the matrix. He had medical credibility with the care providers, yet at the same time was able to function as an advocate of the service side of the matrix.

Such capabilities were not directly and explicitly built into the community management system. Thus, when the scales were knocked off balance by the changing external financial pressures, managerial response and readjustment of the scales became piecemeal and sequential. Each crisis was dealt with individually rather than as a multidimensional problem requiring a number of balancing acts to adjust all the scales at once.

In early 1977 the balance was shifting along one axis of the matrix, that of service orientation. The service orientation is increasingly narrowly defined in terms of quantity of care in response to environmental pressures. As a result, decision-making authority and pressure from management strengthen the nonprofessional authority structure, stressing scheduling, budgeting, personnel utilization over quality, professional development, and clinical support. The result of the pressure ironically has not been to increase quantity significantly but rather to increase resistance by discipline.

If we now review Davis' conditions for the use of a matrix, we observe that MLK does not meet several of them. The first two criteria have been met—balancing discipline and service needs and enriched information processing capacity. The other conditions have not been met in recent months.

As we will see in the next chapter, the information, planning, and control systems do not operate along the different dimensions of the structure. In the ideal matrix structure, equal emphasis would be placed on systems to ensure discipline (quality and human resource development emphasis) as on quantity and administration concerns. At MLK, however, the information and control systems are copied after a functional (discipline-dominated) organization, creating decompositional pressures. Teams do not receive feedback on performance as a unit. Instead, individuals get feedback in comparison to members of their own discipline. Information and control systems are utilized to catch exceptions and to punish, not to initiate problem solving. Productivity data are examined primarily in discipline groups, and not at the unit and team levels. The push is to get more out of the physicians, more out of nurse practitioners. To be successful the matrix needs pressure along both axes. This means focusing more on team output, not individual practitioner's output.

Failure to Think Matrix

The matrix thrives on ambiguity, conflict, and complexity. It is a design that calls for negotiated management. As Paul Lawrence and Jay Lorsch (1969) point out, an important set of variables for organizational effectiveness is the ". . . behavior patterns used to manage intergroup conflict. As individuals with different points of view attempt to attain unity of effort, conflicts inevitably arise. How well the organization succeeds in achieving integration, therefore, depends to a great extent on how the individuals resolve their conflicts." They go on to point out that, "If conflict is to be managed effectively, this influence must be concentrated at the point in the various group hierarchies where the knowledge to reach such decisions exists" (p. 14).

This is not the case at MLK. Neither top nor middle managers show much evidence of thinking matrix. There is little collaborative, open negotiation of differences. The managerial style is one in which directives are generally passed down from above. Information, however, is concentrated in the lower level groups.

Effective matrix thinking would lead one to expect to see a great deal of conflict resolution occurring among professional supervisors representing different points of view, as well as among discipline and unit managers. As of now, unit managers often operate as routine schedulers and more like foremen than as problem-solving, conflict-handling managers. At present these unit managers are not able to operate the matrix design effectively. Furthermore, the discipline groups have become defensive units, protecting their members against pressure for more production and against layoffs and staff cuts.

IMPLICATIONS FOR REDESIGN

In early 1977, MLK management began to return to thinking and behaving matrix. The task facing MLK, as indicated previously, is to make adjustments in a number of major areas all at once. In order to do this, apropriate individuals have to be brought together, conflicting interests, values, and pressures clearly identified, and solutions proposed, negotiated, and decided upon.

In early 1977, the chiefs of the medical disciplines (pediatrics, internal medicine, nursing, and family health workers) began meeting regularly with top management. This occurred for the first time since MLK became a matrix organization. Prior to this, the discipline chiefs met separately but not with the top group. Finally, some of the right people are being brought together. This group possesses most of the necessary information and represents the constituencies needed to arrive at more effective decisions. One group not involved early in 1977 is the unit managers.

A new negotiated order will require making adjustments in each of the four levels of organizational functioning. Examples of the types of adjustments called for in each level are presented in Table 7.1

WHAT A PROPERLY FUNCTIONING MATRIX CAN ACHIEVE TODAY (1977)

Steady State Operations

A properly functioning matrix structure at MLK would foster improved steady state operation. It would provide a way of balancing the demands for quantiy and quality of care. A more efficient deployment of human resources could also be made. By carefully analyzing the service needs of designated population groups, along with the financial constraints imposed by reimbursement realities, decisions could be made regarding the appropriate service mix for each team, that is, the amount of pediatric care, amount of obstetrical care, and so on. This might vary from team to team as their populations vary.

Once the service mix is determined, the matrix provides a rational process for allocating provider capability to teams (how many specialists of each type needed). This matching to demand can be readjusted periodically as environment, patient population size, and service needs change. For example, the deployment of pediatric capability can be adjusted from team to team, depending on the needs of particular patient populations. Some teams may operate without any full-time pediatricians.

The other area needing redesign in the steady state category is its information and control system. Currently these systems are not helping both sides of the matrix to function smoothly. The discipline side needs development as does the information system. A properly operating information system would deal with the team as the unit of production and accountability.

Repair Operations

This level of organizational functioning is most facilitated by the matrix structure. The matrix was initially selected because of MLK's high task uncertainty, incorporating conflicting demands and a resulting high need for repair function. The matrix structure facilitates repair operation because it provides equal weight to conflicting yet legitimate orientations. Thus it legitimizes bargaining activities of team members with unit managers and chiefs of disciplines. For example, when a problem occurs in the area of quality of care received by a particular family (such as improper medication due to a lost medical record), both the chief of the discipline and the unit manager become parties to the repair operation. The matrix facilitates their coming together.

At present, the information and control systems at MLK do not facilitate repair operations. This is due to the fact that, as currently utilized, both the quantity data and the quality of care control system attempt to pick up errors and point out problems. When an error is made, staff members are warned not to repeat it. In other words, information is not used for creative problem solving or to provide positive feedback to individuals. This is especially true in the quality area where only mistakes are fed back. There is never feedback on improvement or good work. Needless to say, a more effective repair operation would be encouraged by making the system less afraid to take risks.

Innovative Operations

The matrix structure currently is a neutral factor for environmental scanning, that is, keeping up with new developments of innovative operation. The environmental scanning operation is discipline oriented. For example, when new developments occur in pediatrics, internal medicine, or nursing, members of those disciplines are made aware of them. The matrix structure neither helps nor hinders the process of keeping up with new developments in the disciplines. The matrix might, in fact, hinder it to some extent.

This is in obvious contrast with a totally discipline-dominated health system. In such a system, there is more interaction among colleagues from the same discipline, hence more chance for informal sharing of new knowledge. However, when it comes to deciding on the implementation of innovations, the matrix structure has an advantage over the discipline system in encouraging a higher quality of decision as well as higher commitment to implementation by different organizational constituencies. The matrix increases the opportunity for bargaining and problem-solving activities that must occur to reach a joint decision.

The negative aspect of the matrix structure for innovation operation is that joint decisions made by different constituencies and conflicting orientations require a large input of time and effort.

It is clear that MLK needs to develop several new structures for innovation. The boundary-spanning networks, people appropriately linked to outside sources of new information, which provide the organization with strategic information are largely underdeveloped. No organization member is currently (1977) responsible for the monitoring of developments in key environmental domains, such as HEW, state and city health agencies, economic trends, health legislation, and so on. Even where there are good boundary-spanning networks, such as some of the links of some of the physicians to various national professional groups, there are no mechanisms for systematically using any of the strategic information obtained to guide important organizational decisions.

This is not uncommon in many organizations. For example, John Hutchinson indicated for multinational firms that

> Organizations can encourage innovation to surface if they provide a supportive climate and structure. Actually much of the organization structure should be compatible with the development of innovations. But very few firms take the time needed to set up structures appropriate to the development of latent talents (1976, p. 52).

In recent years, MLK has not allocated the time to set up such a structure. Even though MLK cannot justify a complex and expensive structure, some key elements need to be built into the organization. The key elements include building top group's capacity to acquire strategic information relevant to its mission; engaging in strategic planning and developing the ability to cope and deal with multiple publics; developing the capability to establish objectives and ascertain that strategies are implemented; and providing proper structure and motivation of employees.

The uncertainty in carrying out these tasks is extremely high. Therefore, the demand for information processing capacity is also high, requiring a very organic design at the top (Galbraith, 1973; Tushman and Nadler, 1976).

Self-Renewal Operations

MLK lacks specific organizational structures and mechanisms for self-renewal operation. The structure discussed for innovative operation above is also appropriate to stimulate more self-renewal operations at MLK. In addition, organizational rewards need to be adjusted to facilitate self-renewal operations at lower levels in the organization, such as among unit managers.

8

ORGANIZATIONAL
PROCESSES

INTRODUCTION

Problem solving, decision making, and control are core processes of a complex organization. It is these processes that make the sociotechnical arrangements and people dynamic. Work is accomplished when people begin to problem solve and to make decisions, whether it be deciding on a simple routine problem or planning the long-range strategy of the organization. Control, then, is seeing that decisions are appropriately carried out.

This chapter sets out to examine the development of problem solving, decision making, and control processes at MLK. The analysis will distinguish between processes dealing with the clinical aspects of the work and those dealing with the administrative aspects. Obviously such a distinction is not always easy to make, but for the purposes of analysis it provides a useful means for better understanding of these processes. The clinical category includes all those activities that directly relate to patient care, such as diagnosis and treatment activities, patient flow and referral activities, patient information system, and the quantity and quality of care provided. The administrative category includes such activities as budgeting, billing, personnel, accounting, purchasing, and inventory, as well as the management information system.

Discussions of problem solving and decision making are treated as one process in this analysis. The process involves thought and action culminating in choice behavior. For example, the decision to treat a hypertension patient with certain drugs instead of attempting to alter his lifestyle is both a decison-making and a problem-solving situation in which there are the following elements: formulation, alternative generation, and information processing. There is little value in attempting to unravel the conceptual distinctions between problem solving and decision making. Whether or not one is an outgrowth of the other has not yet been resolved in the literature, even after 40 years of work (MacCrimmon and Taylor, 1976).

In Chapter 7 a four-level framework was introduced for analyzing organizational functioning (see Table 7.1). This same framework provides the basis for assessing the development of organizational processes at MLK. Table 8.1 presents a summary of the characteristrics of effective problem-solving and decision-making processes and management information and control systems for each level of organizational functioning. The normative, prescriptive statements in Table 8.1 derive from formulations in the management and organization behavior literature. The characteristics of effective problem solving and decision making were drawn largely from the work of Andre Delbecq (1967), Victor Vroom and D.W. Yetton (1973), and Kenneth MacCrimmon and Donald Taylor (1976). The management information and control system characteristics were drawn from Laurence Hrebiniak's (1977) and Edward Lawler's (1976) review of the organization literature on control.

Problem Solving and Decision Making

Table 8.1 differentiates the characteristics of problem solving and decision making for each level. Steady state operation decisions are characterized as programmable, requiring few resources, occurring when time is scarce and the goals and means are clear, such as when decisions are made about how to register new patients, how to bill a patient, or what is to be included in the annual physical exam.

At the second level, repair operation, problems and decisions come in three forms. Form 1, an analyzable type problem, that is, a problem that has a clear and predetermined solution, such as when a patient does not show up for an appointment the schedule is automatically readjusted, or when a bill is not paid a system automatically follows up. Form 2, an analyzable problem, where there are no predetermined solutions, such as in the clinical area when a patient has a unique set of medical and psychosocial symptoms or in the administrative area when the total computerized billing system breaks down. In both cases a unique solution is called for.

Form 3, bargaining conflict type problems and decisions, is that which involves at least two parties with different goals, such as a conflict between union and management or between family health workers and nurses about patient education.

Innovative operation is the third level. Problems and decisions are characterized by lack of clarity about the goals and the means, and often by incomplete problem definition and the lack of alternative solutions. An example might be a decision to integrate a totally new line of mental health services into MLK, or the decision to develop a mixed prepaid and fee for service financial system.

At the fourth level, self-renewal operation, decisions are characterized by being unstructured and self-analytic. An example would be conducting an organizational study with feedback to all members in the organization to initiate an organization development effort.

Table 8.1 indicates that for each level of problem solving and decision making there are appropriate ways of structuring work groups and assigning roles as well as appropriate group climate (Delbecq, 1967). In the final section of this chapter, MLK in 1977 is evaluated in terms of the degree to which these characteristics are found in the organization, both in the clinical area and the administrative area.

Information and Control Systems

In reality these systems are integrally tied into decision making, as they often provide the stimulus for identifying a problem as well as the data for working on a problem. However, for the purposes of the analysis, these systems are treated separately. Table 8.1 identifies the characteristics of information and control systems that facilitate the four levels of operation.

The topic of control will focus on how MLK managed the following (Hrebiniak, 1977): insuring consistency of performance toward common goals; regulating quantity of output; measuring, correcting, and rewarding performance; regulating the quality of the output; limiting discretion or, alternatively, developing clear instrumental relationships in a job or role; and regulating organizational assets.

A basic distinction will be made between elements of control that are error-avoiding and those that are error-embracing. Table 8.2 summarizes some of the differences between the two. The error-avoiding control system is characterized by top-down control with an emphasis on predictability and correctness. The response on the part of organization members is typically one of resistance, low trust, and ritualistic behavior. The error-embracing control system is characterized by an emphasis on self-control, is less constraining, and supports risk taking. The response to such a control system is typically realistic and encourages higher levels of trust (Argyris, 1971; Hrebiniak, 1977).

TABLE 8.1

Organizational Processes and Levels of Functioning

Level of Organization Function	Characteristics of Effectiveness			Management Information and Control System
	Problem Solving and Decision Making			
	Attributes of decision and/or problem	Group structure and rules appropriate	Appropriate group climate	Attributes of system
Steady state operation	Programmable Few resources needed Time scarce Goals and means clear	Automatic (made by system or individual) Interact and communicate for information only Use standard operating procedures, hierarchy and goal setting	Acceptance of the legitimacy for system and/or individual to make decision	Cheap, simple, self-monitoring Rewards desired behavior
Repair operation	Type a: Analyzable type problem (similar to steady state)			Timely catching of mistakes Provides data for correcting mistakes Rewards corrective action, minimizes punishment Provides means to learn from mistakes
	Type b: Unanalyzable type problem	Multiple resources brought together, formal problem-solving procedures followed	Support for creative solutions, compromising	
	Type c: Bargaining conflict	Representativeness of factions, formal procedures	Desire to reach accord Conflict confronting	

| Innovative operation | Goals and means often not known
Incomplete problem definition and lack of alternative solutions | Search procedures for finding alternatives
Leader facilitates creativity and participation
Mixture of expertise | Open, exploring, supports creativity
Consensus oriented | Identifies and monitors new ideas
Provides data from problems as input to stimulate innovation.
Rewards new ideas, especially successful implementation of innovation |
| Self-renewal operation | Unstructured
Self-analytic | Participative involvement of all
Structure for "action research": diagnosis, action, evaluation | Openness
Self-critical
Optimism about control over destiny | System diagnostic capability (human and technical)
Rewards for "action research" mode of management |

Source: Andre Delbecq, "The Management of Decision-Making within the Firm: Three Strategies for Three Types of Decision-Making," *Academy of Management Journal* (December 1967): 329–39.

TABLE 8.2

Behavioral Manifestations in Control Systems

Events, Climate, Attitudes	Based On	
	Avoiding Error	Embracing Error
Control	Primarily top-down; reactive or constraining; emphasis on predictability and correctness	Primarily self-control; less constraining; emphasis on learning; few rules
Allege or accuse of an error	No error occurred; it was unimportant, or someone else's fault	Admit the error; examine the causes and learn for future
Emphasis on	Being right; defensibility of action	Risk taking; innovation
Acceptance of responsibility	Ritualistic	Realistic; shared
Goal setting	Top-down; monocratic; stability of goals (Type A); goals are set standards	Shared; norm that goals must constantly be revised (Type Z); goals reflect conditions which are constantly changing
Decision making	Emphasis on analytical; less concern with intuitive	Emphasis on intuitive, creative; less concern with analytical
Perceptions of power/authority	Fixed pie	Power expansion and sharing
Faced with uncertainty	Avoidance; seek out controllable situation	Confrontation; seek out uncertainty
Attitude toward change	Resistance	Embracing change as necessary
Interpersonal orientation	Guarded; low trust; others are enemies; social Darwinism and Machiavellianism; alienation	Open; less or no concern with enemies; higher levels of trust and helping attitude; psychological involvement
Assumption regarding man	Man-machine model; Theory X; little emphasis on responsibility; "infant" end of continuum	Sociotechnical systems; Theory Y; emphasis on responsibility; "adult" end of continuum

Source: Lawrence Hrebiniak, *Complex Organizations* (St. Paul, Minn.: West Publishing, 1977).

There are problems with each kind of control system. The error-embracing system is extremely costly and difficult to implement and requires very committed people. The managerial trade-off is to decide when one type of system is appropriate. This will be kept in mind as MLK's control systems are analyzed.

Organizational Trade-offs

The significant balancing scales for management and the organization in this chapter are:

1. Quality of the decision versus the commitment of individuals to decision implementation. There are times when these two demands are mutually exclusive, for example, when all the information for a quality decision rests with a few experts. Yet the workers who must implement the decision will be resistant unless they feel that they actually made the decision.
2. Quality of the decision versus time utilization (quickness of decision). These two demands are usually in conflict whenever there is a complex problem with limited resources available. For example, designing patient flow system could take months before an optimum decision. However, the opening of a new clinic might be delayed by this, necessitating a quicker and suboptimum decision.
3. Commitment to the decision versus time utilization (how quickly the decision is made). The most effective mechanism for generating a high level of commitment to decision implementation is to involve those who will be affected by the decision in making it. The greater the level of involvement, the more time is consumed. A balance must be struck between these competing demands.
4. Error-avoiding versus error-embracing control systems. The degree to which the control systems are geared toward catching and punishing mistakes versus the degree to which they are geared toward using data about errors for organizational learning and improvement.

ORGANIZATIONAL PROCESSES
IN PHASE I: 1966–70

The early years of MLK's operation were the high-energy creative years where problem solving and decision making were carried out in an extremely fluid and informal manner. The original core group centered around Dr. Wise would meet at any time and place to discuss issues and problems. They all spent long hours on their jobs. It was not unusual for a member to receive a call from Dr. Wise at 1:00 a.m. to discuss a problem or idea. The group did not stop work at 5 o'clock. Instead, it often had meals together and engaged in informal work discussion through the evening. Such processes are not uncommon in predominantly normative organizations where there tends to be a high degree of overlap for "relationships and groups which fulfill both instrumental and expressive needs" (Tichy, 1973, p. 20).

These years were dominated by activities at the innovative operation level of functioning. Problems and decisions were often not well defined, goals and means were unclear, and a high premium was placed on innovation and new ideas and solutions. The other three levels of organizational functioning were virtually nonexistent in the first couple of years. There was no steady state operation, nothing was routine, and even when some decisions and problems became routine there were few systems, either clinical or administrative, to support steady state operation. At the repair level there were plenty of examples of problems and decisions requiring corrective action; however, as with steady state, there were no systems or procedures in place to help improve operations at this level. Self-renewal operation was valued but not systematically attended to in this phase.

Clinical Decison Making

In the early years of MLK's operation, teams were established by assigning members and giving them a rather nebulous charge—to provide comprehensive health care. Problem solving and decision making were quite informal. They emerged out of the interaction of team members trying to develop ways of handling decisions in the following areas: evaluation of patient health; diagnosis of health problems; treatment of health problems; strategies for recruiting new patients; strategies for educating patients; application of clinical knowledge, such as disease treatment, to the specific patient population; work plans and scheduling of team members; and group conferences for sharing information.

Typically team members reverted to patterns of behavior learned for similar decisions in other work settings. This often resulted in the physician taking control, as he had been trained to do. The result was often that other team members cried "foul" and went to Wise, asking for intervention so that the teams would function more like the ideal they all espoused in which there was true interdisciplinary collaboration without physician dominance.

Problem-solving and decision-making difficulties in the early years were to a large extent attributed to the orientations people brought with them when they joined the team. This is highlighted in an analysis of team problems at MLK by the staff in the 1970 annual report:

> We have attempted to meld together into a smoothly integrated and interdepending unit, personnel with widely disparate backgrounds.

The physicians characteristically are trained in a hospital setting to be individual entrepreneurs. This training constantly reemphasizes ultimate responsibility for everything from lab work to complex diagnosis decisions, and the value system rewards the MD who takes nothing for granted, performs all procedures personally, and assumes total responsibility for all aspects of care. This is not the ideal individual to pick as a member of an interdependent, trusting, multidisciplinary team. The physician's approach to the delegation of responsibility is frequently all or none. He will on occasion maintain responsibility for, and therefore fail to delegate, the performance of many mundane tasks. In contrast, when persuaded or prompted to delegate, he will often do so totally, in effect disclaiming all responsibility for the outcome of this delegation. The professional nurse, whose training classically emphasized her "handmaiden" role vis-a-vis the physician, naturally reacts to this all-or-none attitude ambivalently. On the one hand they are angry over the perceived lack of trust when the M.D. is unwilling to delegate, and on the other hand, they are overwhelmed by the sense of total legal and personal responsibility when he does do so, and in effect washes his hands of the matter. Change in this area is slowly occurring, but will be hastened by improvement in nurse practitioner training, standing orders, and the joint training of health personnel on teams. . . .

Added to this already difficult situation is the position of the Family Health Worker (FHW). The FHW is the only member of the team who is trained with the idea of team care in mind. She brings to the team great understanding of the community, the needs and social milieu of the patient, and is frequently most frustrated by the failure of team function. As the person with the least formal training on the team, she is at an obvious disadvantage in a situation where we proclaim her importance as a resource, and as an equal with other members. . . (MLK, 1970, pp. 60–61).

In another portion of the same report it was concluded that: ". . . recognition of this problem in team coordination is widespread and universally very frustrating. Team conferences are viewed by many of the staff members as useless exercises, if not potentially destructive confrontations."

The difficult experiences in these early years were eventually countered by serious efforts on the part of key MLK staff to develop improved clinical problem-solving and decision-making procedures. These procedures were an effort to develop systems to facilitate steady state and repair operation.

The efforts can be divided into two general areas. One is the development of standard medical protocols dealing with a variety of health and psychosocial problems. The existence of standard protocols provides a mechanism for encouraging more team collaboration and countering some of the effects of the non-team-oriented training of physicians and nurses. The protocols define prescribed approaches to common illnesses and provide guidelines for physicians, nurses, and family health workers. They include "(1) the data base required for patients with the disease, (2) the minimum note required on each encounter concerning the disease, and (3) the broad goals of therapy" (Smith, 1974).

By 1970 MLK had protocols for handling some common primary care problems. The real development in this area, however, did not come about until about a year later in Phase II of MLK's development when the problem-oriented medical records system as well as a quality of care system were actually being implemented. A committee to plan for the use of the problem-oriented medical record system was established in 1968.

The second area in which efforts were initiated to improve clinical problem solving and decision making was the retraining and orienting of health professionals to team work. Again, it was not until the next phase of MLK's development that any sustained effort and systematic work was done in this area, but there was a clear recognition of the need to address ways of orienting physicians and nurses to collaborate.

The lack of procedures for routine (steady state) clinical problem solving and decision making alluded to above resulted in poor utilization of staff and inefficiencies. These were captured in an observational study of physicians that found:

> ... specialists in internal medicine doing the following in addition to the usual tasks which can be done only by the physician: blood pressure readings, diet instruction, calling patients, looking for missing instruments, continuation sheets, disposition sheets, consultation forms, calling and looking for missing charts, X-rays, lab reports, taking a history without an interpreter when the patient can't speak English very well, calling Montefiore in attempt to gain the admission of a patient, doing internal examinations without the medical assistant, receiving calls from patients for refills, side effects, etc. and so on. . . . (MLK, 1970, p. 72)

Administrative Problem Solving and Decision Making

In the early years it had already been indicated several times that administratively MLK was run on a very informal, albeit intense, involvement basis. There were no internally developed administrative procedures for budgeting, personnel, purchasing, and so on. Thus, as in the clinical area, there were no systems to facilitate steady state and repair operations. The only formal systems or procedures that existed were those either carried out by Montefiore or imposed by OEO for auditing and accounting purposes. In general, administrative decisions were made by Wise or, as MLK grew in size, by members of the core group who were informally given control over different areas of activity.

As in the clinical area, the lack of procedures and guidelines for administrative decision making began to create problems and frustrations by the end of the start-up period. By 1970 MLK management had started to take steps in the direction of developing basic accounting, personnel, and information capability.

Control Systems

In both the clinical and administrative areas, control was either based on professional socialization, that is, internal reliance on the self-control of professionals who, through their training and socialization, had internalized certain norms and patterns of behavior, reducing the need for monitoring them on the part of the organization; or informal direct interaction among workers, that is, control was exercised by members of the staff interacting with each other and correcting, monitoring, and so on. Often the informal control came in the form of confrontation after something went wrong (repair operation).

On the positive side, the general tenor of the control system was "error embracing." People were encouraged to learn from mistakes and to take risks. Everyone was learning together. The control process encouraged innovative operation. By the end of this phase, Montefiore was beginning to work with MLK in the design and development of control systems in the administrative area—accounting, inventory, billing, purchasing, personnel, and so on—primarily to facilitate steady state operations.

ORGANIZATIONAL PROCESSES IN PHASE II: 1970–74

This period witnessed the development of most of the MLK systems in the clinical and administrative areas. These included both problem-solving and decision-making systems as well as control systems. This phase was what Greiner (1972) characterized as the "direction" phase, during which the organization develops accounting systems for inventory and purchasing; incentives, budgets, and work standards; more formal communication and hierarchy of titles and positions; and lower level supervisors treated more as functional specialists than as autonomous decision-making managers.

In contrast to the previous phase of MLK's development, steady state operation activities dominated the scene. Tremendous managerial and organizational energy and resources went into developing new systems and procedures in both the administrative and clinical areas. By the end of this phase, MLK had a new form of medical rewards, quantity and quality of care systems, billing, accounting, and personnel systems.

Clinical Problem Solving and Decision Making

In 1970 the problems that were plaguing health teams were having a negative impact on the quality of decision, the commitment of team members both to carrying out decisions and to the concept of working on a health team, and the effective utilization of team personnel. One team stated that, "we react to crises rather than planning; we never decided what the team should be doing; there are differing priorities—medical, social, agency, building; very little time for joint planning" (MLK, 1970).

The MIT group in 1969 and 1970 focused heavily on decision making and problem solving, the areas that this group found to be most critically deficient. The team development work of the MIT group focused on helping the teams address the following issues (Beckhard, 1974, p. 73):

1. Which members perform which work?
2. How will this be decided?
3. What problems of patient identification, diagnosis, treatment, health maintenance and patient education need to be dealt with by the team working as a group?
4. What information is needed from one member by another? For example, what does the pediatrician, who sees the patient in his office, need to know from the family health worker, who visits the family at home, about the life style, values, and living conditions of the patient's family?
5. What pesonal and professional development needs does each member have? How can team help meet these needs?

The result of the MIT team development work was that, by 1971, teams at MLK began to function more effectively. There were higher levels of collaboration and more participation in decision making. The first two criteria of team effectiveness—quality of decision and commitment to the decisions—showed marked improvement. Time utilization was not as important then because of ample financial and manpower resources in the system. Even though the MIT development strategy was designed to help the team decide when to use collaboration and when not to use it, and to only involve team members who had relevant information in the decisions, the actual result was different. The strategy tended to push teams toward collaborative and participative decision making when at times it was not needed for a quality decision and the cost in time and energy could not be justified. In other words, in the absence of strong pressure for quantity of care, the overcollaborative team approach was acceptable.

Perhaps even more important than the team development work was the simultaneous development of medical protocols coupled with instituting the problem-oriented medical record (POMR). The POMR system developed by Dr. Lawrence Weed reorganizes the record "to encourage the production of a logical and complete document relating to the patient's problems. A problem list serves as the table of contents or index to the rest of the information contained in the record" (Reed, 1974, p. 181).

The POMR consists of four elements: (1) Data base—development of a patient profile. (2) Problem list—based on information in data base. A list of problems is coupled (can be medical, social, or psychiatric), analyzed together, and listed on the front of the record. (3) Initial plan—what is to be done related to each problem. (4) Progress note—includes subjective data, objective data, and assessment of the plan (SOAP) for each problem. The POMR approach has the following advantages (Weed, 1974a, p. 182):

1. Problems can be treated in relation to other problems.
2. Important facts are readily available so problems can be treated easily.
3. Table of contents by problem makes tracking problems easy.
4. Encourages better coordination among practitioners as methods and plans are clearly laid out on the chart.
5. Family care can be encouraged as a link can be established between a family problem list and an individual's list.

It took several years for MLK to implement the POMR. A pilot study was launched to train one team in its use. The implementation was difficult, as the physician and nurse had to relearn procedures they had been using for years. The difficulty in implementing the new system was evident when after a year trying the POMR (in 1971) there were still "lists in only one third of the charts in the sampling but two thirds of the charts contained the SOAP (subjective data, objective data, assessment and plan) format, to some degree" (Reed, 1974).

Along with the POMR system was the development of the protocols. These were developed primarily to guide the quality of care on the teams. An important secondary gain in developing these protocols was that issues of how teams solve problems and make decisions had to be explicitly dealt with. This is because the protocols include identifying the responsibilities of team members for different aspects of many primary care problems. Protocols were developed for pediatrics, internal medicine, venereal disease, ob-gyn, and adult care (see Appendix C for a more detailed description of the POMR, protocol development, and chart review at MLK).

By the end of this phase, 1973, MLK had systems in place that greatly enhanced problem solving and decision making for team delivery of care. It is quite evident that improved team problem solving and decision making at MLK were dependent on both the development of the POMR and protocols as well as specific team development activities organized by the MIT group. Neither approach would have been sufficient. Some of these same systems, as we shall see, provide the basis for the clinical control system at MLK.

Clinical Control Systems

Control in the clinical area is two-faceted. On the one hand there is productivity control as reflected in the quantity of work (number of patients) and, on the other hand, there is the quality of care (reflected in adherence to protocols).

Quantity of Care

A system was developed in Phase II to collect data on how many patients each practitioner (nurse, physician, dentist, family health worker) sees for each session. This information is reported on a monthly basis, with total number of patients seen for the month, the average per session, as well as the average number of times a patient is seen by each provider. The data are used by management to identify individuals not meeting production norms (each provider group has an average number of patients per session target). The information system is most congruent with steady state operations, that is, it facilitates consistency of performance within provider groups and regulates the quantity of output.

Quality of Care

MLK developed a very extensive medical audit system during this phase (see Appendix C for the description). Practitioners regularly engage in a random chart review in which diagnoses and health plans are reviewed. One problem with the review is that it is not utilized for anything other than catching mistakes. It therefore fulfills steady state operation needs and some repair needs, but does not help manage the unstructured repair operations, or innovative operation. It is basically error avoiding.

These systems took several years to develop and implement. By 1974 they were all in operation and had a profound impact on improving clinical problem solving and decision making and controlling the quantity and quality of work. The greatest impact was on steady state and repair operations; little attention was given to ongoing mechanisms for supporting innovative and self-renewal operations.

Administrative Systems

The 1970–74 period was also the time when MLK developed its own internal capability for accounting, billing, purchasing, and inventory, as well as its own computer system to support both administrative and clinical activities. The development of these systems was accomplished through a large infusion of help from Montefiore. At MLK, Edward Martin coordinated the development of these systems. (See Appendix D for descriptions of MLK administrative systems.)

PHASE III: 1974–PRESENT

In contrast to the two previous phases, Phase III did not have any one level of organizational functioning that dominated. The steady state operation systems were mostly all developed by 1974, thus only minor tinkering and readjustments have been made since. There has been a decline in innovative operation as MLK has faced a situation of tighter resources.

The most significant shift during this phase, however, has been the aforementioned shift in environmental pressure. The result is that pressure exists internally that either exacerbated problems that were always present and part of the procedures and system or led to new ones. The final section of this chapter assesses these problems.

1977 ASSESSMENT OF ORGANIZATIONAL PROCESSES AT MLK

One consistent theme throughout this book is that MLK entered a major transition period in 1977. This is reflected in mounting organizational strains at all levels and is no less apparent with regard to organizational processes. Table 7.1 identified some of the current (1977) conditions at MLK as well as implications for change. This chapter concludes with a further assessment of organizational processes at MLK at each level of organizational functioning.

Steady State Operation

In 1977 steady state clinical decision making and control at MLK were in need of several readjustments. This was so even though the basic systems—patient information, patient flow, protocols, and so on—were well designed and supported the delivery of high quality primary care. The readjustments called for were (1) Decision making: Restructure the teams to reflect more efficient use of multiple disciplines (see Chapter 6 for framework to guide this effort, Table 6.2). Balance quantity and quality considerations reflected in the matrix (discipline quality input and administrative quantity input). (2) Control: Control system used solely to catch quality errors and catch those not meeting "quotas," therefore error avoiding and in need of redesign so as to encourage and reinforce good performance. Focused on individual providers, not on team; need new control system to measure control team performance as well as individual (both quantity and quality).

The steady state administrative decision and control processes were generally adequate in 1977 and only minor readjustments were called for. One such readjustment was the financial system at MLK. The system is geared toward external controls—HEW, Medicaid, and other third-party payers, as well as Montefiore. Each of these external agencies has need for financial data. These needs, however, usually result in aggregating data in such a fashion that it is not helpful for internal management control.

Internal financial systems are only partially utilized. Each unit has a budget, but one that it feels is based on what it got last year adjusted to projected financial conditions for the new year. The budgeting system is not tied to systematic planning throughout the system. If it were, then some form of marketing would be carried out to determine population needs and demand and then service mix would be reexamined and adjusted with careful assessment of cost. The balancing of the market and financial needs is based on precedent. No real financial accountability is felt by units, as they do not feel they really have a plan and that their budgets are used for accountability purposes. The potential is high for using the financial systems as stimulation for more innovative operations. This might be accomplished by turning each unit into a responsibility center with accountability for its own financial viability. This would have to be carefully weighed against the potential for dysfunctional interunit competition.

Repair Operation

The second level of operation, repair, was in greater need of adjustment than the steady state operation. This was due to the problem identified in Chapter 7, which indicated that the matrix structure was never adequately implemented at MLK. Repair problems and decisions in the clinical area were characterized by avoidance of conflict between discipline groups on the team; conflicts between quantity pressures and quality pressures unmanaged; and lack of matrix type managerial behavior (little explicit conflict management and bargaining). To respond to these problems MLK could reinforce the matrix structure for guiding problem solving, that is, recognize the legitimacy and utility of conflicting points of view; and encourage open conflict management, especially among middle- and top-level managers.

The clinical control systems at MLK have already been characterized as error avoiding. For effective repair operation they need to be tilted toward the error-embracing end of the scale. This can be accomplished by a major control system redesign effort involving organization members at all levels (see Tables 8.1 and 8.2 for design criteria).

An example of a relatively simple control system change is to alter the way in which the random chart review process is utilized. This could be accomplished by having individual practitioners and teams collaboratively establish quality targets that they monitor not only to catch mistakes but to improve care constantly. An altered system could become the mechanism for stimulating improvement in health services and the source of new service innovations by using the information as a stimulus to provide review and problem solving rather than a narrowly defined management tool for picking up mistakes.

In addition there are other quality measures that are not being collected, such as hospital utilization. This is strategic if MLK's strategic plan over the next five years leads it in the direction of prepaid services. In a prepaid system hospital utilization is the key to financial viability and also a good long-term indicator of quality of care. Thus, it would not be a bad idea to start collecting information and building a control system that monitors hospital utilization rates for providers and for teams.

Another quality indicator that is not part of the MLK system is a breakdown of services provided each month by provider, by team, and by specialty group. This information helps both quantity of care and quality of care. It can be keyed to cost and revenue data. It can also provide a way to monitor patient needs for various services to see whether the service mix provided matches what is needed by the patients. Over- or underutilization of services would be readily apparent.

In the administrative area some of the same problems found in the clinical area are manifest. There are inadequate procedures for managing conflict; therefore a need exists for both new decision-making mechanisms and supporting control systems.

Innovative Operation

The innovative operation level at MLK in 1977 was organizationally unmanaged. No formal structure existed for systematically linking the organization to sources of new ideas and knowledge, nor were there mechanisms for translating new ideas and knowledge into practice. In the clinical area new innovations occurred because individual practitioners or the chiefs of discipline groups discovered something new and introduced it to others. This process was occurring less and less, as there was little organizational support for it. The same was true in the administrative area, where no systematic management and/or organization development activities were occurring.

The implication is that for MLK to stimulate innovative operation, two conditions must be met. First, a structure and set of processes are needed for monitoring new ideas and knowledge. This means seeing that key people are encouraged to keep up in their fields, attend continuing education programs, and so on. Second, there should be mechanisms for incorporating new ideas, such as in-service training, management help, and support for incorporating new practices and procedures. MLK needs practices and procedures. MLK needs to develop a systematic research and development capability.

Self-Renewal Operation

The fourth level of operation, self-renewal, has also been dormant at MLK from 1974 to 1977. In 1977, however, the need for MLK to begin to develop a long-term strategy was apparent. The top management group was reconstituted to include the medical discipline chiefs and was starting to problem solve the future course for MLK. In addition to top-level strategic planning, self-renewal activities are called for at lower levels in the organization; however, such efforts should build on a clear strategic plan from the top.

9

MLK'S ACCOMPLISHMENTS AND THE FUTURE

INTRODUCTION

The year 1977 marked the end of a decade of operation for MLK. The prognosis for the next decade is highly uncertain. As identified in each of the previous chapters, the decade was a major transition point for MLK. This chapter outlines some of the major accomplishments by MLK in its first decade as seen by the author and by six individuals who played significant roles in the growth and development of MLK. These same individuals did some future gazing and identified major hopes and fears for the future of MLK. The final section of this chapter presents a proposal for helping an organization such as MLK make a successful transition.

ACCOMPLISHMENTS

Chapter 1 listed some of MLK's accomplishments as seen by the author. We will now return to an examination of MLK's accomplishments as seen by the six individuals personally interviewed in late 1976 and early 1977. They were asked to identify the most significant accomplishment for MLK. The individuals were David Kindig, M.D., director of Montefiore Hospital and Medical Center, who did part of his residency at MLK, 1970–71, and was medical director at MLK in 1971; Gloria Perry, R.N., director of Bathgate satellite, MLK, former director of training, who worked as community public health nurse in community prior to start of MLK; Deloris Smith, MPH, director of MLK, who started at MLK in first group of family health workers; Harold Wise, M.D., founder and director of MLK, 1966–70; George Silver, M.D., professor, Yale University, formerly of Montefiore's social medicine department, then a deputy at OEO during the early years of the neighborhood health center; Mo Katz, deputy director, Montefiore Hospital and Medical Center, who has had major responsibility for managing Montefiore's relationship with MLK, especially since 1974.

The major accomplishments reported by them were training of community people (from service area) for meaningful jobs in the health field; providing high level services for a population that had none or inadequate services; and the use of nonphysician type people in the provision of health care (including involving family members). As Deloris Smith indicated:

> I guess it would be the opportunity to explore the possibilities of using non-physician type people to provide health care . . . that we actively seek out other people to provide care that we feel does not require the technology of a highly trained physician but could be done by somebody else . . . we've even used the household members to help. . . . I think that this piece of information will be helpful in trying to cut overall cost by way of National Health Insurance. You can use people who are not overly trained, therefore, you can pay them a little less and they can still produce very well.

Other accomplishments included the creation of the family health worker role; the OEO philosophy of worrying as much about the patients who don't come through the door as about the ones who do; being an organization where people cared about the quality of personal relations and the quality of work life; as a health facility very successful, yet it did not come near to accomplishing the overly ambitious and unrealistic expectations we had for the neighborhood health center and the community change agent.

Another class of accomplishments not mentioned by the interviewees is the contribution MLK made to primary care management and organization design. My personal list would therefore add the following accomplishments: the development of an internal structure managed by community members; the development of interdisciplinary health care teams with supporting systems—the problem-oriented medical record, protocols; the development of quality of care procedures; the use of a matrix organizational structure to facilitate team functioning; and the use of management and behavioral science knowledge and consultation.

FUTURE HOPES AND FEARS FOR MLK

These accomplishments provide the backdrop for future accomplishments by MLK. The same group of individuals who provided the list of accomplishments produced the following list of hopes for MLK's future: maintain the type of comprehensive services offered (two individuals), hope it will survive as a model (two individuals) not just for "poor" people but for all classes, and be able to adapt and reach out, to become solid.

> I see three things: One is that it will continue to provide care. Second, that it will continue to provide jobs and that we would be able to continue to hire people from that neighborhood and train them, as people move out to other places, and third, of course, the whole business about the governance. I really would hope and I continue to hope that the place could be self-governing. That's something I would very much like to see. And I think it's the one area in which we have failed miserably. I think we have done well in the other two.

One clear theme in the discussion about MLK's future with these six individuals was that of consolidating and maintaining the gains from the first decade in light of worsening financial odds. The shift in MLK's operation in response to new financial realities is expressed by Gloria Perry:

> I think we're working on it. In fact up until a few years ago, we offered all services free and we never asked anyone about any kind of coverage and never insisted on paying any bills. I think it is now time to get reimbursement for some of the services that we do offer which I think means great pride in trying to be self-sufficient. However, with the cost of everything now, I don't know if health services will ever be able to be self-sufficient. . . . I don't know if we'll ever catch up.

This theme is more strongly underscored in the list of fears for MLK's future: that we will be unable to continue to give comprehensive services; that the whole financial picture for primary care is so bleak in New York that MLK will not be underwritten; that the surrounding facility (community) will get so demolished that it won't pay to be here; and that the community board won't have tight enough restrictions and control by HEW (could destroy the organization).

Dr. David Kindig expresses his major fear for MLK in the context of health care financing in New York:

. . . the whole financial arrangements are terrible, you have to worry about just the basic viability of this kind of a program, much less so in the old days when they were underwritten . . . it's not going to be underwritten now. I think that's not even the worst fear; the routine operating fear is how to keep it solvent, doing a good job without a lot of extra money . . . it ties in with the whole financial problem for ambulatory care in general, and the plight of the cities and New York in particular. I don't have special concerns for MLK, I'm worried about the outpatient department, our emergency room [Montefiore], and the city hospital outpatient clinic in the same way.

Finally two others, Dr. George Silver and Dr. Harold Wise, expressed their fears as follows: that because no one in Washington has the guts to stand up and fight for these centers and the services they provide, they will not be allowed to survive; that MLK becomes just another place to work where personal relations and quality-of-life issues become secondary.

Another one of the six, Mo Katz, expressed his fear in the following terms:

What I hope is that they manage to survive until we get national health insurance. Clearly with the health situation in New York City and the likely increased difficulties of Medicaid, and so on, they may have to do things to survive which would be inimical to what the center is all about and they may get themselves reduced more and more into a "Medicaid mill" and that would be a great pity. The problem is can they survive in some other form with or without board control until national health insurance comes, when they can have their future pretty secure.

In 1977 MLK was on the verge of entering a new developmental stage. In order to make the passage successfully and avoid making the previously listed fears come true, it would be necessary to mobilize considerable managerial and organizational resources. The first decade of MLK's development had in effect brought the organization full circle from 1966 when there was a need to develop a clear organizational mission and mandate to 1977 when the original mission and mandate had reached the end of its life cycle and needed to be reformulated.

The irony is that MLK succeeded in being highly successful as the mandate stated in 1966. And this was in part why MLK was in trouble in 1977. It had been successful at being innovative and providing needed health services. This was problematic because, as stated, the ground rules have changed. The prime responsibility for organizations engaged in servicing poverty-area patients, and increasingly any class patients, has now been shifted toward more cost-effective use of financial resources. Maximization of health services has become secondary. This is obviously a very significant shift, causing great organizational uncertainty in regard to mission, strategy, and organizational design.

At the start of 1977, the MLK management was feeling the considerable impact of this uncertainty, yet management was still in flux regarding what to do. Pressure had mounted to a level requiring a new master strategy embodying global change. The Thompson (1967) formula for organization under conditions faced by MLK prescribes an inspirational, entrepreneurial mode of decision making. This would unfortunately be a difficult prescription for an organization in which routinization of charisma (building in legitimate leadership without basing it on the charisma of the founder) and bureaucratization so recently took place.

The alternative to an inspirational mode of decision making based on a charismatic leader would be to mobilize a large-scale self-renewal operation at MLK. This would entail focusing managerial and organizational energies toward diagnosing both environmental trends and organizational strengths and weaknesses. The first task confronting management would be to develop what William Newman (1972) calls a "master strategy which sets the basic purpose of an enterprise in terms of the services it will render to society and the way it will render these services." Newman includes the following components as part of such a master strategy:

1. Establishing the service market niches that are propitious in view of society's needs and the organization's resources [for MLK this would include deciding what services and for whom they should be provided].
2. Selecting the underlying technologies [how to carry out the tasks] and ways of attracting inputs [money and patients].
3. Expressing these plans in terms of targets.
4. Setting up sequences and timing of steps toward these objectives which reflect the organization's capabilities and external conditions [environment] (p. 57).

The master strategy is linked to a management design that is made up of necessary alterations in the sociotechnical arrangement and organizational processes. An outline of a process that MLK could follow is presented in the next section of this chapter.

The proposed action calls for a planning mode of strategy formulation similar to that followed in 1970 when MLK worked with Richard Beckhard and the MIT group. The approach is characterized in Table 3.1 as one in which there is a high faith in the mission; an explicit mission; rational decision making; global change; flexible, elite control with a moderate amount of grass-roots control; and which is proactive.

ORGANIZATIONAL PASSAGE:
A SELF-RENEWAL PLAN FOR MLK

Strategic Assessment

The process is diagrammatically presented in Figure 9.1. The first assessment that should take place is of the environment, now and in the future. The relevant aspects of the environment that influence MLK in the present and those projected to be influential in the future should be carefully mapped. This entails identifying such factors as economic trends relevant to primary care; HEW policy; state, county, and local health financing trends; as well as general economic trends of the region and specifically of the South Bronx.

A sociopolitical analysis on the environment would be undertaken. Included here would be an assessment of the New York Health and Hospital Corporation's intentions for the Bronx; the intention of the director and coordinator of health for New York City;* the views of patients and potential patients toward health care; and the federal government's prospects for National Health Insurance.

Finally, an area study is called for. The demographic trends of the South Bronx would be mapped. Health needs would be determined and the original health survey done in 1966–67 by MLK staff might possibly be redone. A mapping of all actual and potential competitors and/or collaborators in health service should take place, using an approach similar to Evan's (1966) organizational set analysis, which facilitates systematic mapping of interorganizational relations.

The second assessment would be of current organizational strengths and weaknesses (see Figure 9.1). The assessment would include an examination of many of the same organization components discussed in the chapters of this book: organizational design and the health team (Chapter 6), the macroorganization design (Chapter 7), and organizational processes, decision making and problem solving, and control (Chapter 8). The assessment would focus management on the trade-offs identified in each of those chapters and the implications of such problems as the conflict on primary health care teams, the decomposition of the matrix, inadequately developed and differentiated problem-solving and decision-making processes, and the error-avoiding nature of the control systems.

---

*This same individual holds the following positions: health service administrator, chairman of the Health and Hospitals Corporation, chairman of the Interagency Health Council, deputy state health commissioner for New York City, deputy director of the state Health Planning Council and chairman of the executive committee of the New York City Health Systems Agency.

FIGURE 9.1

Strategic Planning Model

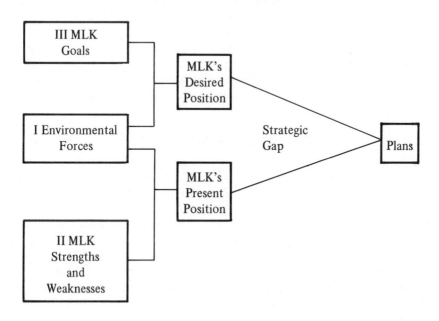

Source: Louis Gerstner, "Can Strategic Planning Pay Off?" *Business Horizons*, December 1972, p. 8.

The environmental assessment and the assessment of organizational strengths and weaknesses would be combined to provide an assessment of current position. This would help MLK focus more systematically on the degree to which its organization is inconsistent with environmental conditions.

The third major assessment is organizational goals, both current and future, within the context of environmental constraints and opportunities. These goals would implicitly incorporate trade-offs between such factors as financial viability and the value of providing needed services, which in some cases are in conflict. MLK's basic position with regard to this issue is grounded in organizational values that stress both provision of services to those in need without regard to ability to pay as well as provision of certain types of nonreimbursable services that MLK deems important for its client population, such as programs dealing with lead-based paint in apartments and school programs.

The dilemma for MLK is the following. Health care financing currently favors acute and chronic disease care, encouraging over-utilization of laboratory tests, x-rays, and so on. But the values fostered at MLK tend to favor preventive care, outreach services, counseling, screening, and child and family development. Future goals should reflect compromise. Hence, the desired position of MLK (Figure 9.1) in the future will be to survive in the realities of health care financing without having to give up too much in the preventive, comprehensive care area. In addition, MLK's strategy should be to stay flexible in the event of changes in health financing brought on by National Health Insurance.

Developing a Strategic Plan

Once the desired position of MLK is developed, then the "strategic gap" is identified (see Figure 9.1). This is the distance between current position and the desired position. The strategic gap is closed by developing a strategic plan, the elements of which are presented in Table 9.1 and Table 9.2. Once the plan is developed, it should be subject to a review process that systematically examines major assumptions reflected in the proposed plan. An example of such a review is presented below. The left column lists the planning assumptions and the right column lists the assessment of assumptions:

Major Assumption in Proposed Plan	Assessment of Assumption
Patient base will increase 10 percent per year	Inconsistent with past three years of declining population
Medicare reimbursement will stay constant	Unlikely. May go down
National Health Insurance will be in effect in three years	Highly uncertain, even if so may not be comprehensive
Inflation will be at 6 percent per year level	Uncertain with Carter's conomic plans
Federal creation of new jobs will benefit MLK by creating a new training department	Uncertain

The proposed plan assumptions (left column) are, by and large, unrealistically optimistic, for example, it is highly unlikely to increase revenues through more registered patients in existing area (population is declining); it is unrealistic to count on National Health Insurance in near future; and federal jobs are unlikely to help MLK. The result of such a review process could be a total revision of the strategic plan based on a new set of planning assumptions. Once planning assumptions are acceptable, the plan is finalized.

TABLE 9.1

Summary of Strategic Plan Elements

Environmental Assessment	Organization's Position
Broad economic assumptions	Statement at mission
Key government regulatory trends	Interrelated set of financial and non-financial objectives
Major technological forces	Statement of key strengths and weaknesses
Significant market opportunities/ threats	Forecast of operations—revenues and cash flow
Explicit strategies for potential competitors	Major future program

Strategic
Options

↓

Alternative Strategies*

↓

Requirements for Implementing
Each Strategy

↓

Contingency Plans

*See Table 9.2 for examples.
Source: Louis Gerstner, "Can Strategic Planning Pay Off?" *Business Horizons*, December 1972, p. 8.

TABLE 9.2

Alternative Strategies

Typical Strategic Issues	Typical Decision Alternatives
Should investment be made to strengthen position in service X?	Commit to $200,000 now, $4 to $5 million over next six years or begin to "milk" or divest service X
Should we provde more outreach delivery of services Y and Z?	Begin to phase out outreach services or signicantly upgrade outreach services
Should we seek new catchment area and develop satellites?	Begin search for new catchment areas or initiate a major study of cost reduction and productivity in existing area and facility

Source: Compiled by the author.

Developmental Needs for the Strategic Plan

Following the strategic plan formulation an assessment of developmental requirements is made. This includes people, financial, technical, and operational considerations. The MLK assessment would focus on required organization design changes at both the team level and the total organization level, changes in organizational processes as well as an assessment of the human resource implications of the plan.

Team Redesign

The key determinant of the health care team design would be the types of health services that MLK decides to offer. The particular mix of health services would be subject to an analysis guided by the framework presented in Table 6.2, which includes a multidimensional analysis of health services: focus of care—individual to community; target of care—from acute medical to preventive psychosocial; and depth of intervention.

Each cell of the Table 6.2 matrix can be examined to help guide decisions regarding how an individual team should be structured to deliver a particular service. This would include determining the appropriate mix of health providers (physicians, nurses, family health workers) required for variable task demands. The team redesign process could be guided by a framework developed by Richard Hackman (1976) that stresses three critical intervention points for improving team effectiveness: design of the group task itself, composition of the group, and performance strategies used by the group in carrying out its work.

Organization Redesign—Macrolevel

Once the health teams, which are the basic work unit at MLK, are redesigned, then attention would be focused at the total organizational sociotechnical arrangement. The core issue at this level is to structure the organization for integration and coordination of effort. The matrix design was a solution at one point in MLK's development. A reassessment of the appropriate organizational form may substantially alter this design. The redesign effort would make adjustments in the structure to facilitate all four levels of functioning: steady state, repair, innovation, and self-renewal.

Organizational Processes

Adjustments in this area were discussed in Chapter 8. They would be made to insure that the redesigned team and organizational design were driven toward accomplishment of the strategic plan. Problem-solving and decision-making processes would undoubtedly be altered at the team level to reflect the variable task demands reflected in team redesign. At an organizational level more emphasis would be placed on differentiating appropriate problem-solving and decision-making processes facilitative of repair, innovative, and self-renewal operations.

The modification of the control processes would focus on moving toward more reliance on error-embracing control systems.

Human Resource Implications

The final step is a human resource, or people assessment. The following steps are involved (Kubicek, 1972):

1. Prepare a human resource inventory to determine who does what, who reports to whom, who has authority and how much.
2. Review the use of the present staff in light of the proposed new strategic plan. For key positions prepare a list of all suitable candidates and their special skills, experience, aptitudes and potential.

3. Ascertain what personnel problems with respect to vested interests would be involved in implementing the plan and develop a plan to deal with it.
4. Determine human resource problem areas, places where necessary resources are not in the organization or where there are surpluses. Decide what to do about problems.

IMPLEMENTATION

The result of the strategic planning process would not be an inflexible mandate for all major MLK activities but rather a scheme for the future with provisions that allow the plan to be modified and adapted over time to a highly uncertain environment. The scheme would provide the guidelines for new service community participation, and administrative strategy at MLK.

10

INTRODUCTION

The MLK case has provided the health care management field with an important social laboratory. MLK was established, along with many other OEO-sponsored organizations, as a demonstration. MLK, like the other demonstrations, should be carefully and systematically analyzed to deepen our understanding of the dynamics of managerial and organizational processes in the primary health care field. This final chapter sets out to summarize the analysis carried out in this book.

As a case history of one neighborhood health center, this study can offer no conclusions about the management and organization design of primary health care organizations. As a case study, however, it can serve as the basis for developing hypotheses that may eventually be shown to have wider application.* Therefore, in this final chapter a set of propositions relevant to primary care and possibly to other organizations is developed. This framework facilitates generalizing from the MLK case and provides a guide for future research efforts (Gouldner, 1954; Georgopoulos and Mann, 1962; Georgopoulos, 1975).

---

*Karl Weick (1969) argues that while case studies have "a richness of detail, they have at least four drawbacks: They are (1) situation specific, (2) ahistorical, (3) tacitly prescriptive and (4) one sided" (p. 18). The MLK case study is vulnerable on all four counts, yet unlike many other case studies it does respond to several of the criticisms. First, it is historical in its focus. Second, it attempts to deal explicitly with any material that is prescriptive rather than have it broadcast subliminally as a tacit message. Finally the case is written with a self-consciousness about trying to avoid being one-sided.

A DEVELOPMENTAL MODEL

Chapter 2 presented an organizational model that provided the categories for the analysis of MLK. The model focused attention on key organization components. Each chapter of the book then examined a component in depth as it developed at MLK. A second model briefly presented in Chapter 2, Greiner's concept of the phases of organizational development, reemerges from the analysis of the MLK case. That is, the analysis of MLK provides us with a developmental model of a health care organization.

The developmental phases that emerged are similar in some respects to Greiner's, yet are sufficiently unique to MLK to require formulation of a new set of developmental phases. The case analysis provides an interesting chronicle of how one primary health organization passed through three major phases of development: (1) a start-up phase, characterized by high levels of creativity and innovation; (2) a system development phase, characterized by a great deal of energy and resources being invested in the design of systems (management and patient) and the organization (bureaucratization); (3) a consolidation and stabilization phase, in which only small incremental changes took place and minor repair operations occurred managerially and organizationally. A fourth self-renewal phase was perched on the horizon in 1977, characterized by major efforts to reformulate organizational strategy and to redesign the organization.

Each phase was dominated by a set of organizational concerns that absorbed most of the managerial energy and organizational resources. The resolution or management of these concerns provided the impetus for pushing the organization on to the next developmental stage. The solutions to problems at one stage were often the cause for problems at the next stage. In accord with Greiner's model (1972), "each phase is both an effect of the previous phase and a cause for the next phase."

The acceptance of a developmental view of organization is in no way inconsistent with perspectives that view other factors as major determinants of organization design and effectiveness. It is recognized and accepted that organization environment may in fact contribute more to determining how the organization develops than historical forces. At this point, however, the relative weight of these factors, environment and history, represents an area with little theoretical guidance and virtually no research guidance. The developmental phases briefly described below are, therefore, discussed as if environmental uncertainty and technology were held constant.

Start-up Phase

New organizations such as MLK often spring into life with a tremendous burst of energy. This is especially true for those that are started with fairly large grants, enabling them to hire immediately large numbers of staff and acquire physical resources prior to providing any services or generating any income. The existence of start-up grants vastly accelerates Phase I.

The major organizational concern of Phase I is the mobilization of people, ideas, and resources around a unifying mission. This is facilitated by an entrepreneurial decision-making mode generally built around a charismatic leader/founder. The process is further facilitated by developing an organizational climate that is experimental, engenders high levels of worker commitment to the mission, and deals openly with differences and conflict. At MLK the leader/founder, Harold Wise, energized groups of people to do "their own thing," to get projects started, to try things out and not to worry about how well they would work out or who would pay for them. The organization was dominated by innovative operations. There were virtually no steady state operations. This was also true of repair operations, which were not systematized.

The more successful the organization is at being innovative, the more difficult it becomes to manage. This was true at MLK due to the increase in size and complexity brought on by the successful implementation of the various innovative projects—job training, community development, health care teams, and so on. The phase ended with the organization facing confusion, destructive conflicts, and frustration.

System Development Phase

The dominant theme during the second phase of development is rationalization and development of managerial practices and procedures to provide a semblance of order from the confusion created in Phase I. The organization makes a heavy investment in steady state operations. The conditions that facilitated development in Phase I—experimenting, creativity, entrepreneurial leadership—actually hinder development at the second phase. The decision-making and leadership facilitative of Phase II development is a planning mode often accompanied with a forceful and driving managerial style. Often, as was the case at MLK, special outside resources and expertise are needed to assist in the design and

development of management systems (the MIT group, Montefiore technical assistance, and so on).

By the end of Phase II, the organization has been driven hard. In the
case of MLK not only were steady state systems being developed but the
community managers were being trained and moved into their new
positions. This phase ended with the organization experiencing a sense of
accomplishment as well as a sense of having had to work hard to achieve
it.

Stabilization and Consolidation Phase

For some organizations this phase may be relatively brief, as it is
simply a time to test the newly designed and implemented systems and to
make minor alterations and improvements. At MLK this phase had added
significance, as it was during this period that the community managers
were first given total responsibility for managing the center. The
dominant organizational activities were repair operations. The emphasis
was on continuity, and both innovative operations and self-renewal
operations were at low levels. The phase comes to an end when a disturbance comes along to put pressure on the organization for change. The
disturbance can be internally generated, such as personnel problems, or,
as is more likely, externally generated, such as the MLK where both
financial pressure and a declining population base are pushing the organization to action. This is the point at which MLK found itself in 1977.

Self-Renewal Phase

An effective organizational response to new disturbances of the
magnitude facing MLK in 1977 is to engage in self-renewal activities that
focus on reformulating the strategy and design of the organization. The
phase is characterized by high levels of activity and a survival-oriented
drive on the part of management. The tension around survival provides
the energy that needs to be constructively channeled. The danger in this
phase is that it tends to pull the organization apart into factions rather
than providing a unifying force. The natural tendency among groups
within the organization faced with a shrinking pie is to try to maintain
their same share. Successful passage through this phase leads the organization into a system redesign and development phase, necessary to implement the new organizational strategies developed in the self-renewal
phase (Tichy and Beckhard, 1976).

GROWTH AND DEVELOPMENT:
CONDITIONS FOR SUCCESSFUL PASSAGE

Organizational passage from one phase of development to the next occurs as a result of the successful balancing of dominant trade-offs found in each phase. The balancing occurs through a combination of environmental forces, developmental forces, and managerial action. The mix of these three forces with regard to their impact on resolving developmental dilemmas varies both among organizations and over time within the same organization. In extreme cases the organization's environment may account for almost all the growth and development, and no matter what management does, good or bad, it can't help or hinder passage from one developmental phase to the next. On the other hand, some organizations require a great deal of managerial balancing of trade-offs to pass from one phase to the next.

MLK falls in the middle. Its environment definitely played a key role independent of developmental forces and managerial action. However, managerial action was also a critical factor in MLK development and was required to help MLK pass from one phase to another. The remainder of the chapter proposes a set of conditions that tend to facilitate organization growth and development in different phases. The conditions are assumed to be important in situations where all three forces—environmental, developmental, and management—play a determinant role. Table 10.1 identifies the conditions proposed for each phase of development for successful passage.

Awareness and understanding of these conditions provide managers with guidelines for focusing their action and resources. It is clear that some of the conditions are out of their control, others partially controlled, and still others totally controlled by them. The manager as juggler and balancer of trade-offs needs to decide which factors to ignore, which to massage gently, which to manipulate, which to activate, and which to try and prevent. The developmental view of organizations proposed in Table 10.1 identifies focal points for each organizational component at each phase of development. The conditions proposed in Table 10.1 apply to the MLK case and can be tentatively proposed for other similar primary health care organizations.

Start-up Phase

The phase starts with a crisis of mission and strategy. The core start-up group often has a vague mission or image of some future organization. There tends to be a high value commitment accompanied

TABLE 10.1

Conditions for Successful Organizational Growth and Development

Organizational Components	Phase I Start-Up	Phase II System Development	Phase III Stabilization	Phase IV Self-Renewal
Environment	Benign supportive internal community control	Pressure for more internal community control	Moderate pressure for internal community control	Strong pressure (either opportunity and/or threat) external community control
Mission/strategy	High commitment	Rationalized explicit	Continuity of strategy with piecemeal changes	Reformable explicitly and rational
Sociotechnical	Adaptive experimental	Rationalized formalization	Stabilized, little change from Phase III	Redesign
Organizational processes	Fluid; commitment over time or quality; error-embracing	Systematized; more of a balance between error-embracing and avoiding	Routinized; error avoiding dominant	Redesign
People	Innovators; idealistic	Pushers in charge	Good followers needed	Innovators and pushers needed
Emergent networks	Extensive internal and external social linkages	Supportive of management efforts	Variety of social networks	Reenergize to support the top

Source: Compiled by the author.

by strong interpersonal and social bonds among the core group, but no clear mission and an even less clear strategy.

Successful resolution of this crisis and passage through this phase are not likely if there is a high level of environmental uncertainty, lack of charismatic leadership, and little organizational fluidity. To facilitate start-up the environment should provide a benign if not supportive context. Given these environmental conditions, management action and resources are facilitative during this phase to the extent they encourage multiple innovative projects that mobilize creative, innovative individuals to be entrepreneurial; and give people their freedom and room to run.

The focal scales that emerge during this phase are:

Mission/strategy: tilt toward high commitment.
Sociotechnical arrangements: tilt toward the adaptive and experimental.
Organizational processes: tilt toward being fluid, commitment more important than the quality or the speed with which decisions made, and control systems are error-embracing.
People: tilt toward innovators and idealistic types.
Emergent networks: tilt toward far-reaching ideological homogeneous internal and external networks.

The phase ends with a crisis of confusion, frustration, and ambivalence toward the charismatic leadership.

System Development Phase

The confusion, frustration, and ambivalence crisis does not tend to get resolved unless pressure comes from both the environment and internally for taking managerial action. Without the pressure the organization tends to continue to flounder. In MLK's case, individuals such as Dr. David Kindig, Dr. Edward Martin, and Professor Richard Beckhard were the major conduits for external pressure, each telegraphing the message that the ship was not in good order. The resolution of the crisis is facilitated by managerial focus on rationalization of mission and strategy and system design, development, and implementation.

The scales that became focal during this phase are:

Environment: balance begins shifting to put performance pressure on the organization, internal community control dominates.
Mission/strategy: balance shifts to rationalized and formalized design, emphasis on steady state operations.
Sociotechnical arrangements: balance shifts to rationalized and formalized design, emphasis on steady state operations.
Organizational processes: balance shifts to systemization, and more emphasis on avoiding errors, maintaining regularity.

People: balance shifts from innovators to pragmatic pushers and doers.

Emergent networks: balance shifts to less extensive and less ideological networks to those that are directly supportive of management's system development task.

The system development phase results in reducing confusion, frustration, and ambivalence, yet it creates a new crisis, the crisis of control, centralization, and cynicism about management. Even though the new crisis is often accompanied by a sense of accomplishment, the organization has been pushed and power has become more centralized, resulting in a reaction against control and a cynicism about management. Often a greater we/they dynamic between managers and workers sets in.

Stabilization/Consolidation Phase

For organizations such as MLK that not only developed new systems but a totally new group of managers in the preceding phase, the stabilization and consolidation phase is critical. The organization requires time to take a rest and be able to make adjustments in the newly developed systems. The crisis of control and centralization tends to be a dominant theme through this phase and may not be resolved prior to the onset of new crises and passage to another phase. Management action facilitative of successful passage through this phase is characterized as testing and modifying new systems and testing and modifying managerial behavior and effectiveness.

The scales that are most central during this phase are:

Environment: balance continues to shift toward more pressure for efficiency and internal community control dominates.

Mission/strategy: balance does not shift, the theme is continuity of strategy with any changes being piecemeal.

Sociotechnical arrangements: stabilized, little shifting.

Organizational processes: balance shifts toward more rationalized and more error-avoiding control systems.

People: balance shifts toward doers and less toward innovators and leaders.

Emergent networks: balance shifts toward less instrumental and more toward friendship and social networks.

A new crisis is likely to emerge during this phase, the crisis of complacency. The organization can become lazy, timid, and unable to mobilize itself for either innovative activities or for self-renewal activities.

It is as a result of some pressure, generally rather severe environmental pressure, that the crisis of complacency can give way to a crisis of survival. The crisis of survival tends to mobilize energy to propel the organization into the next phase, self-renewal.

Self-Renewal Phase

Passage into this phase is in response to an extreme external pressure (either an opportunity or a threat). With MLK it was a threat that forced it to mobilize around survival issues. The managerial response facilitative of this phase is mapping the environmental pressures, reformulating mission and strategy, and mobilizing the organization for action around redesign and change of strategy (Beckhard, 1974).

As Chapter 9 briefly outlines, passage through this phase tends to require a high level of managerial activity and resources. The phase concludes with a redirected, redesigned organization ready to pass into another phase of stabilization and consolidation. If this successfully occurs at MLK, it will have made its passage from innovation to self-renewal.

Effective passage from phase to phase, a healthy developmental process, is measured in terms of how well the organization meets the conditions of health, as cited by Edgar Schein:

1. Ability to take in and communicate information reliably and validly.
2. Internal flexibility and creativity to make the changes which are demanded by the information obtained.
3. Integration and commitment to the goals of the organization, from which comes the willingness to change.
4. An internal climate of support and freedom from threat, since being threatened undermines good communication, reduces flexibility and stimulates self-protection (1970, p. 126).

From a managerial and organizational behavior perspective, the recognition of strong developmental forces in organizations provides a promising avenue for future research. Such research is especially relevant for the one major growth area in the health field, primary health care, where there will continue to be the start-up and development of new organizations.

Similar analyses of other health care organizations are needed to determine how unique the MLK experience was. In the meantime, the scales and trade-offs identified as key in this final chapter deserve both managerial and research attention.

CONCLUSION

The case of MLK chronicles how a predominantly normative organization developed into a mixed, more complex normative and utilitarian organization, thus requiring a system with controls based on both intrinsic values and extrinsic, economic rewards. The development was fraught with dilemmas and trade-offs, some of which were unique to MLK and others more general in nature.

INTRODUCTION

The case study of MLK is categorized as a field study that Zelditch (1969) indicates "is not a single method of gathering a single kind of information." Field studies utilize multiple methods to study people in situ (Scott, 1965). The field study method was employed in such classic investigations as Phillip Selznick's (1949) study of the TVA, Alvin Gouldner's (1954) study of a gypsum company, Seymour Lipset et al.'s (1956) study of the International Typographical Union, Melville Dalton's (1959) study of managers, and Leonard Sayles' (1958) study of factory workers. In each case, a variety of methods, such as participant observation, structured observations, interviews, questionnaires, and document analysis, were employed. The MLK study also employed multiple methods. The criteria for method selection should be "the nature of the phenomena under investigation and the objectives of the study which must determine what approaches are taken and what material are gathered by what methods" (Scott, 1965, p. 262).

Before the methods used in the MLK analysis are discussed, a number of dilemmas facing field studies in general are identified and discussed in relation to the MLK study.

Demands of Scientific Colleagues Versus Demands of Subject Groups

As Scott (1965) points out, the researcher is a member of a scientific community that values "the importance of knowledge for its own sake, and is subject to norms, such as the need to approach his subject with detachment and objectivity." On the other hand, the subject group may not share these values; even if they do they will have an additional set of demands, namely, to get something worthwhile out of being studied. The two sets of demands can easily become conflicting and mutually exclusive, resulting in the researcher being thrown out of the organization under investigation or the researcher losing any sense of detachment and objectivity.

The author's involvement with MLK waxed and waned between these two extremes. In the early years, 1972–73, the author was primarily a researcher with detachment. However, there was a period, 1974–75, when the author was a consultant to both the top-management group and the board, and was thus deeply involved in the organization. This phase was followed by a more detached period, 1976–77, as a researcher during which the sifting and sorting for this study took place.

The experience of being deeply involved with the management group and others within MLK provided insights and understandings that would not have been possible as a detached researcher. As a direct participant in managerial and board activities, I was able personally to experience some of the difficulties of managing a few of the trade-offs and scales discussed in the study. By standing back and analyzing the total MLK experience, I feel I was able to regain some of the advantages of being an objective researcher with the added benefit of some firsthand experience working with management and the board.

Participant Versus Observer Dilemma

As Scott (1965) points out, the longer one wants to stay involved in an organization as a researcher, the greater the pressure to be a participant. This was true at MLK, and, as discussed in the researcher versus subject group dilemma, I ended up becoming highly involved as a participant.

Exploratory Versus Descriptive and/or Hypothesis Testing

In the case of MLK, there was no dilemma. The study was clearly an exploratory study. As such, it is an in-depth analysis of one organization over an extended period of time aimed at developing insights and hypotheses for future research. There were no hypotheses to be validated; there was, however, an interesting and complex organization undergoing a great deal of change that called for greater understanding.

PHASE I OF THE STUDY

My involvement began in 1972. This phase was characterized by involvement as a detached researcher. In 1972 I became involved with MLK via work with interns and residents in social medicine at Montefiore who participated in training sessions designed to provide them with team skills for more effective participation on the MLK teams. Richard

Beckhard was the one who involved me in this training activity. At the same time, he began to tell me about MLK and its importance as a prototype health organization. In the spring of 1973, Richard Beckhard and I co-taught a course on organization development at Columbia in which about six staff from MLK were students. By the end of spring, I had heard enough about MLK to be convinced that Beckhard was correct about its importance and I decided to launch an organizational study of MLK.

In the summer of 1973, I organized an action research project for MLK that was to involve interviewing, questionnaire data, and feedback to the total organization. I presented my idea to Deloris Smith and Edward Martin, who agreed to coopeate. My initial reasons for launching the study were to learn more about health organizations and to involve a group of Ph.D. students in a field study. For MLK, they saw the study as an opportunity to learn more about themselves and about organization development, specifically about the use of survey feedback interventions.

Interviews

To start the process, the Columbia team, in early fall of 1973, interviewed a random sample of 60 staff members to determine their perceptions of problems at MLK, their perceptions of the goals of MLK, how they managed their work, their views of the future of MLK, and their assessment of the decision-making processes at MLK. The responses from these interviews provided the basis for developing a paper-and-pencil questionnaire (see Attachment 1) that was administered to 234 MLK staff (60 percent).

Questionnaire

The questionnaire results were summarized and fed back to all groups in the organization from top to bottom. The feedback process was designed to energize staff to solve problems identified by the survey. There were a total of 12 half-day feedback meetings all conducted by the author. These included top management, middle management, X-ray department, pharmacy, laboratory, housekeeping, and Units 1 through 5.

The outcome of the feedback process was varied. Some groups mobilized themselves to engage in improvement projects, while others never followed up the feedback meetings at all. The top- and middle-management groups met for a day-long meeting with Richard Beckhard as consultant to begin work on problems in communication and administration uncovered by the survey.

PHASE II OF THE STUDY

In the summer of 1974, June Tayler and I conducted interviews with all the top managers at MLK, as well as with Harold Wise and Mo Katz, about the development of the community management system. These interviews and documents (OEO proposals and annual reports) provided the data for Chapters 4 and 5 (see Attachment 2 for interview guide).

Late in 1974, the top-management group at MLK decided to begin working to improve its own team effectiveness and to plan for the future. Deloris Smith contacted me and asked if I would be available and willing to work with the top group. I said yes. In preparation for a weekend workshop with the top group, I interviewed each of its members regarding current organizational problems and how they were working as a management group. The weekend workshop provided me with an intense involvement with the top-management group. The weekend was followed up with several meetings at MLK to work on long-term goals for MLK.

The final set of activities in Phase II was my work with the community board. During the summer of 1975, Mo Katz, deputy director of Montefiore, contacted me to request that I help train the community board to assume grant responsibility. I worked with the board for several meetings, including a weekend workshop discussed in Chapter 5. The work with the board never resulted in any substantial movement toward board takeover of the grant, but afforded me a first-hand experience with all of the board members and a better understanding of the political dynamics of the board in 1974.

Through this phase, I was keeping field notes on my experience with MLK. In addition to the above activities, I was still training the interns and residents in social medicine to work on health teams.

PHASE III OF THE STUDY

The final phase of my involvement in the field study of MLK cycled back to a more detached researcher mode of involvement.

Interviews

I conducted interviews with key figures in MLK's development to determine what they perceived to be the major accomplishments of MLK and their future hopes and fears for MLK. These interviews were discussed and the list of individuals interviewed is found in Chapter 9. In addition to these inverviews, I conducted informal interviews throughout this period with key informants at MLK about various aspects of organizational functioning and events that were taking place.

Questionnaire

In the summer of 1976, David Nadler and I engaged MLK in another questionnaire study. The study was of the incentive and control system at MLK as related to health providers. Attachment 3 is a sample questionnaire that was filled out by 17 physicians, 9 dentists, 8 nurses, 30 family health workers, 17 medical assistants, and 9 dental assistants. These data were not systematically analyzed and used for the case analysis of MLK but did provide supportive material used in Chapter 8 on organizational processes.

Documents

The most useful of all the documents used in this case study were the annual reports. There were six annual reports for MLK covering the years through 1973. The annual reports were unique documents, as they were extremely candid, self-analytic reports that were generally written by staff from all areas of MLK. The annual reports also included special studies on the neighborhood and topics such as family health care. Other documents relied upon included the management information system reports, OEO proposals, memos, special research reports, and HEW documents on MLK.

ATTACHMENT 1   ID Number:

_____

DR. MARTIN LUTHER KING, JR. HEALTH CENTER
ACTION RESEARCH STUDY

This questionnaire has been designed to help MLK plan for the future. C.1
The study is being carried out by a group from Columbia University in 1-3/
collaboration with several MLK staff members. Please help MLK by   4/
answering *ALL* questions to the best of your ability. Most questions 5-6/
require only circling a number. If the questions do not say things the way
you would like to say them, please circle the response that comes closest
to your own opinion. Feel free to add comments either in the margin or
at the end of the questionnaire.

A code number has been placed on the first page of the questionnaire; this number coincides with your name. Only the Columbia group
will ever have access to names and numbers; no member of the MLK staff
can relate your name to the questionnaire.

Some questions ask you to give us the names of other people. Their
names will be assigned code numbers, so that individuals won't be
identified.

The results of the study wil be made available to *all* MLK staff
members in such a way that individuals will not be identifiable.

YOUR RESPONSES ARE TOTALLY CONFIDENTIAL.

* * *

Instructions

1. *MOST QUESTIONS CAN BE ANSWERED BY CIRCLING ONE OF THE NUMBERS PROVIDED OR FILLING IN AN ANSWER SPACE. IF YOU DO NOT FIND THE EXACT ANSWER TO FIT YOUR CASE, USE THE ONE THAT IS CLOSEST TO IT.*
2. PLEASE ANSWER *ALL* QUESTIONS IN ORDER.
3. REMEMBER, THE VALUE OF THE STUDY DEPENDS UPON YOUR BEING STRAIGHTFORWARD IN ANSWERING THIS QUESTIONNAIRE. YOU WILL *NOT* BE IDENTIFIED WITH YOUR ANSWERS.

* * *

SECTION I

FOR EACH STATEMENT BELOW, INDICATE TO WHAT EXTENT YOU FEEL THE STATEMENT IS TRUE OF THE MARTIN LUTHER KING, JR. HEALTH CENTER (MLK). Please *CIRCLE THE NUMBER* to indicate your answer.

	To a very little extent	To a little extent	To some extent	To a great extent	To a very great extent	
1. To what extent are you told what you need to know to do your job in the best possible way?	1	2	3	4	5	7/
2. To what extent do you feel your pay is related to how well you perform your work at MLK?	1	2	3	4	5	8/
3. When decisions are being made at MLK, to what extent are the persons affected asked for their ideas?	1	2	3	4	5	9/
4. People at all levels in this Center may have information about how to do things better. To what extent do you feel such information at all levels is used?	1	2	3	4	5	10/

5. How are differences and disagreements between departments (areas) handled at MLK? *Circle* the *one* that is most typical.
   1. Disagreements are almost always ignored.
   2. Disagreements are *often* ignored.
   3. Sometimes disagreements are accepted and worked through; sometimes they are ignored.

4. Disagreements are usually accepted as necessary and desirable and worked through.

5. Disagreements are almost always accepted as necessary and desirable and are worked through.   11/

6. How are objectives set at MLK? Circle *one*.

1. Goals are announced with no chance to raise questions or give comments.

2. Goals are announced and explained, and chance is given to ask questions.

3. Goals are made up, but are discussed with workers and sometimes changed before being used.

4. Different alternative goals are made up by management and people are asked to discuss them and say which they think is best.

5. Problems are presented to those people who are involved, and the goals felt to be best are then set by workers and management together.   12/

READ THE CATEGORIES ON THE RIGHT CAREFULLY, THEN ANSWER EACH OF THE QUESTIONS BELOW. *Circle* the number to indicate your answer.

	Very Dis-satis-fied	Some-what Dis-satis-fied	Neither satis-fied nor Dis-satis-fied	Fairly sat-is-fied	Very sat-is-fied	
7. All in all, how satisfied are you with the persons in your workgroup?	1	2	3	4	5	13/
8. All in all, how satisfied are you with your immediate supervisor?	1	2	3	4	5	14/
9. All in all, how satisfied are you with your job?	1	2	3	4	5	15/
10. How satisfied do you feel with the progress you have made in this Center *up to now*?	1	2	3	4	5	16/
11. How satisfied do you feel with your chances for getting ahead at MLK *in the future*?	1	2	3	4	5	17/
12. All in all, how satisfied are you with middle management at MLK?	1	2	3	4	5	18/
13. All in all, how satisfied are you with top management at MLK?	1	2	3	4	5	19/
14. All in all, how satisfied are you with the union at MLK?	1	2	3	4	5	20/

	Very Dissatisfied	Somewhat Dissatisfied	Neither satisfied nor Dissatisfied	Fairly satisfied	Very satisfied	
15. How satisfied to you feel with the types of health services given at MLK?	1	2	3	4	5	21/
16. How satisfied are you with the quality of health care given at MLK?	1	2	3	4	5	22/
17. In general, how satisfied do you feel patients are with MLK?	1	2	3	4	5	23/

WRITE THE NAME OF YOUR SUPERVISOR IN THIS SPACE: 24/26
(for professional staff this does *NOT* mean your professional supervisor).
ANSWER QUESTIONS 18 THROUGH 23 ABOUT THE PERSON YOU IDENTIFIED.

READ THE CATEGORIES ON THE RIGHT CAREFULLY, THEN ANSWER EACH OF THE QUESTIONS BELOW. Please *CIRCLE* the number to indicate your answers.	To a very little extent	To a little extent	To some extent	To a great extent	To a very great extent	
18. To what extent do you feel your supervisor has confidence and trust in you?	1	2	3	4	5	27/
19. To what extent do you have confidence and trust in your supervisor?	1	2	3	4	5	28/

HOW MUCH DOES YOUR SUPERVISOR NEED EACH OF THE FOLLOWING TO BE A BETTER MANAGER? Please *CIRCLE THE NUMBER* to indicate answer.

	To a very little extent	To a little extent	To some extent	To a great extent	To a very great extent	
20. More information about how her/his people see and feel about things.	1	2	3	4	5	29/

	To a very little extent	To a little extent	To some extent	To a great extent	To a very great extent	
21. A work situation that lets her/him do what she/he already knows how to do and wants to do.	1	2	3	4	5	30/
22. More interest in and concern for people who work for her/him:	1	2	3	4	5	31/
23. More information about principles of good management.	1	2	3	4	5	32/

IN THE QUESTIONS BELOW, *WORK GROUP* MEANS ALL PERSONS WHO REPORT TO YOUR SUPERVISOR. *CIRCLE THE NUMBER* to indicate your answer.

24. To what extent are persons in your work group willing to listen to your problems?						
(1) This is how it is *now*:	1	2	3	4	5	33/
(2) How I'd *like* it to be:	1	2	3	4	5	34/
25. To what extent do persons in your work group maintain high standards of performance?						
(1) This is how it is *now*:	1	2	3	4	5	35/
(2) How I'd *like* it to be:	1	2	3	4	5	36/

IN THE QUESTIONS BELOW, *WORK GROUP* MEANS ALL PERSONS WHO REPORT TO YOUR SUPERVISOR. *CIRCLE NUMBER* to indicate your answer.

26. To what extent do persons in your work group offer each other new ideas for solving job-related problems?						
(1) This is how it is *now*:	1	2	3	4	5	37/
(2) How I'd *like* it to be:	1	2	3	4	5	38/
27. How much do persons in your work group encourage each other to work as a team?						
(1) This is how it is *now*:	1	2	3	4	5	39/
(2) How I'd *like* it to be:	1	2	3	4	5	40/

	To a very little extent	To a little extent	To some extent	To a great extent	To a very great extent	
28. To what extent does your work group make good decisions and solve problems well?						
(1) This is how it is *now*:	1	2	3	4	5	41/
(2) How I'd *like* it to be:	1	2	3	4	5	42/
29. To what extent do persons in your work group know what their jobs are and know how to do them well?	1	2	3	4	5	43/
30. To what extent do you have confidence and trust in the persons in your work group?	1	2	3	4	5	44/
31. To what extent are the equipment and facilities you have to do your work with adequate, efficient and well maintained?	1	2	3	4	5	45/

THE FOLLOWING QUESTIONS REFER TO THE 1199 STRIKE WHICH TOOK PLACE IN NOVEMBER. Please CIRCLE number to indicate your answer.

	To a very great extent	To a great extent	To some extent	To a little extent	To a very little extent or not at all	
32. Did you feel the 1199 strike in New York was appropriate?	1	2	3	4	5	46/
33. To what extent were you satisfied with the performance of top management during the strike?	1	2	3	4	5	47/
34. To what extent were you satisfied with the performance of the union delegates at MLK during the strike?	1	2	3	4	5	48/

	To a very great extent	To a great extent	To some extent	To a little extent	To a very little extent or not at all	
35. To what extent do you feel the MLK union delegates represented their members well?	1	2	3	4	5	49/
36. To what extent did the strike unite MLK staff members?	1	2	3	4	5	50/

37. During an average day at MLK, who are the people you *most often* interact with? (Please PRINT last name, then first initial.)

NAME

Person I interact with:
a. most _____ 51-53
b. second most _____ 54-56
c. third most _____ 57-59
d. fourth most _____ 60-62

SECTION II
PROBLEMS AT THE MARTIN LUTHER KING, JR. HEALTH CENTER

Here is a list of some possible problems at MLK. For each problem, check how much you feel it bothers *you personally*. Please *CIRCLE THE NUMBER* which indicates your answer.

	Bothers me very much	Bothers me somewhat	Bothers me very little	Not a problem to me	
1. Patients do not come for appointments on time.	1	2	3	4	63/
2. The possibility of future budget cuts.	1	2	3	4	64/
3. Lack of clarity concerning how decisions are made about the allocation of resources (money, staff facilities).	1	2	3	4	65/
4. Power struggles among staff members.	1	2	3	4	66/
5. Racial issues among staff members.	1	2	3	4	67/

	Both-ers me very much	Both-ers me some-what	Both-ers me very little	Not a prob-lem to me	
6. Not enough management know-how to run the center if Dr. Martin leaves.	1	2	3	4	68/
7. Poor communication among people I work with on a daily basis.	1	2	3	4	69/
8. Poor upward communication at MLK.	1	2	3	4	70/
9. Poor communication down from top management.	1	2	3	4	71/
10. Lack of clear guidelines for carrying out jobs.	1	2	3	4	72/
11. Not enough resources—staff, facilities, etc.—to provide quality health care to large numbers of people.	1	2	3	4	73/
12. Too much pressure for quantity of care; not enough for quality of care	1	2	3	4	74/
13. Too many meetings; not enough time to get work done.	1	2	3	4	75/
14. The possibility of the community advisory board taking over the administration of the HEW grant from Montefiore.	1	2	3	4	76/
15. Too much paper work and bureaucratic "red tape."	1	2	3	4	77/
16. Inadequate medical record system.	1	2	3	4	78/
17. Lack of long-range future planning at MLK.	1	2	3	4	79/
18. Other (specify)					
_____ _____	1	2	3	4	80/

Begin CARD #2

19. Of the problems listed on the preceding page and this page, which ONE bothers you the MOST? Write the number (for example, 01, 02, 03, etc.) of the problem here:

_____   7-8/

20. Of the problems listed on the preceding page and on this page, which ONE bothers you SECOND most? Write number here:

_____   9-10/

Think about the problem you just listed that bothers you the *MOST*.
Who at MLK have you spoken to recently about that problem? List the
names of the people you most often speak to about this problem (first,
second, third most).

Person I speak with about this problem:

most_____	11-13/
second most _____	14-16/
third most _____	17-19/

Advisory Board

How likely do you feel that the present Community Advisory Board will take
over administration of the HEW grant from Montefiore? Circle one number.

1 very likely	4 neutral—don't know
2 quite likely	5 somewhat unlikely
3 somewhat likely	6 quite unlikely
	7 very unlikely 20/

Circle one number

25. If the present community board were in charge of MLK's funds, how
    would you feel?

1 strongly in favor	5 slightly opposed
2 moderately in favor	6 moderately opposed
3 slightly in favor	7 strongly opposed 21/
4 neither in favor nor opposed	

26. If the present community advisory board were in charge of MLK, do
    you feel that certain groups of workers would be favored over certain
    other groups of workers?

    1 very likely to favor one group over another
    2 quite likely to favor one group over another
    3 somewhat likely to favor one group over another
    4 somewhat unlikely to favor one group over another
    5 quite unlikely to favor one group over another
    6 very unlikely to favor one group over another   22/

27. Do you feel the present advisory board is representative of the
    community?

    1 Yes, very representative of the community
    2 Yes, somewhat representative of the community
    3 No, not representative of the community   23/

28. Are you in favor of having some sort of community advisory board?
    1 strongly in favor   5 slightly opposed
    2 moderately in favor   6 moderately opposed
    3 slightly in favor   7 strongly opposed
    4 neither in favor nor opposed   24/

29. If there is a community advisory board, which of the following groups
    should have members on the board? (Circle as many as apply)
    1 MLK staff
    2 MLK patients
    3 Local community leaders who are not patients
    4 Local community members who are not patients   25-28/

30. Which of the following groups is it most important to have
    represented on the board? (Circle one)
    1 MLK staff
    2 MLK patients
    3 Local community leaders who are not patients
    4 Local community members who are not patients   29/

SECTION III

GOALS

THE FOLLOWING IS A LIST OF POSSIBLE GOALS FOR THE MARTIN LUTHER KING, JR. HEALTH CENTER. THEY HAVE BEEN SUGGESTED BY A VARIETY OF PEOPLE AND REPRESENT DIFFERENT CONCEPTIONS OF THE FUNCTIONS OF MLK. FOR EACH STATEMENT INDICATE HOW IMPORTANT THE GOAL IS TO MLK NOW BY PUTTING A CIRCLE AROUND THE APPROPRIATE NUMBER.

	How important a goal is it *now*:				
	very impor- tant	moder- ately impor- tant	slightly impor- tant	not impor- tant at all	
01. To provide jobs for community residents	1	2	3	4	30/
02. To provide training for jobs inside and outside of the center for community members.	1	2	3	4	31/
03. To deliver comprehensive family-oriented, health care.	1	2	3	4	32/

	very impor- tant	moder- ately impor- tant	slightly impor- tant	not impor- tant at all	
04. To expand with new programs and services.	1	2	3	4	33/
05. To give the community control of health care.	1	2	3	4	34/
06. To help patients deal more effectively with their environ- ment and society.	1	2	3	4	35/
07. To be an advocate for com- munity members in areas other than direct health care, such as housing, etc.	1	2	3	4	36/
08. To become a self-sufficient, independent organization without federal aid.	1	2	3	4	37/
09. To be an organization which functions like "one big happy family."	1	2	3	4	38/
10. To provide the best quality care even at the cost of less quantity	1	2	3	4	39/
11. To provide the most care for the most people even if quality suffers somewhat.	1	2	3	4	40/
12. To participate in developing new comprehensive health care programs.	1	2	3	4	41/
13. To do research on health services	1	2	3	4	42/
14. Other (specify)					
_____	1	2	3	4	43/

15. Of all the goals listed on the preceding page and this page, which *TWO* are most important?

The *most* important is:_____
(list number) 44-45

The *second* most important is: _____
(list number) 46-47

SECTION IV

FUTURE HOPES FOR THE MARTIN LUTHER KING, JR. HEALTH CENTER

BELOW IS A LIST OF POSSIBLE FUTURE GOALS FOR MLK. READ THEM OVER AND THEN ANSWER THE QUESTIONS AT THE BOTTOM OF THE PAGE.

01. To serve greater numbers of patients.
02. To become controlled by a community board.
03. To provide jobs and training for community members in the Center.
04. To provide more community and social services.
05. To be self-sufficient and not require federal funding.
06. To be an organization that functions like one big happy family.
07. To provide opportunities for staff of MLK to get training and move up to higher level jobs.
08. To get more involved in preventive health care in schools and the community.
09. To develop the primary health care team approach more.
10. To increase the number of physician specialists to provide more specialist health services.
11. To improve cost effectiveness and serve more patients with the same size staff.
12. To provide better quality care.
13. Other (specify) ——————————————————————

* * *

16. MOST IMPORTANT GOAL
    Of all the goals listed above, which ONE do you personally feel is the most important for MLK to strive for.
    WRITE NUMBER OF THE GOAL HERE: _____   48-49/
17. WHAT I'D SACRIFICE TO ACCOMPLISH THE MOST IMPORTANT GOAL
    If you had to GIVE UP two other goals to accomplish the goal you just listed, what would they be?   50-51/
    WRITE NUMBER OF TWO GOALS HERE:_____ _____ 52-53/
18. SECOND MOST IMPORTANT GOAL
    Which goal do you personally feel is the second most important for MLK to try and achieve.
    WRITE NUMBER OF THE GOAL HERE: _____   54-55/

19.   WHAT I'D SACRIFICE TO ACCOMPLISH THE SECOND MOST
     IMPORTANT GOAL
     If you had to give up *another two* goals, what would they be?
     (Do not indicate same answer you gave in question 17.)
              WRITE NUMBERS OF TWO GOALS HERE: 56-57/
                           _____   _____ 58-59/

20.   Think of all the people you personally speak with at MLK about the
     future of MLK. List the three people who you *personally* speak
     to who you find to have the best ideas about the future of MLK:
     (Please PRINT).
     1. _____   60-62/
     2. _____   63-65/
     3. _____   66-68/

SECTION V

PRESENT-DAY DECISIONS AT MLK

*IN ORDER TO UNDERSTAND HOW MLK WORKS, WE NEED TO
FIND OUT HOW DIFFERENT KINDS OF DECISIONS ARE MADE.
IN THIS SECTION WE WILL ASK YOU TO NAME PEOPLE WHO
INFLUENCE IMPORTANT DECISIONS AT MLK.*

1. What three persons do you consider to have the most say about hiring,
     firing, and promoting in your department, e.g., health services, admin-
     istration, training, and allied health services? (Include yourself if you
     feel you are among the top three.) Please PRINT.
                         NAME
     (1)   The MOST influential person is: _____ 69-71/
     (2)   The SECOND MOST influential person is: _____ 72-74/
     (3)   The THIRD MOST influential person is: _____ 75-77/

Begin Card #3

2. What three persons at MLK do you consider to be most influential in
     making decisions about the quantity, quality, and type of health care
     delivered at the Center? (Include yourself if you feel you are among the
     top three.) Please PRINT.
         Name THREE people: (1) _____ 07-09/
                           (2) _____ 10-12/
                           (3) _____ 13-15/

3. What three persons at MLK do you consider to be most influential regarding the future of MLK? (Include yourself if you feel you are among the top three.) Please PRINT.

Name THREE people: (1) _____ 16-18/
(2) _____ 19-21/
(3) _____ 22-24/

PEOPLE WHO MOST INFLUENCE MY WORK

4. Think back over the past month. Now consider all the people in your area both at your level and at other levels. Think about the people who you personally speak to who would be most likely to influence you in work matters—that is, people whose opinions and advice you would both seek and respect. List these people in order, starting with the name of the person whose advice and opinion would, in general, be of most value to you. Please PRINT.

The MOST influential person is: _____ 25-27/
The SECOND MOST influential person is: _____ 28-30/
THIRD MOST influential person is: _____ 31-33/

SECTION VI

BACKGROUND INFORMATION

1. What was your age at your last birthday? _____ 34-35/
2. What was your place of birth? _____ 36-37/
3. What is the highest level of schooling you have had? Circle.

1 8th Grade or Less   5 Completed College
2 Some High School   6 Some Graduate Work
3 Completed High School   7 Completed Graduate or
4 Some College   Medical School   38/

4. Sex: 1 Male 2 Female   39/

5. Are you:
1 Single   3 Widowed
2 Married   4 Divorced or separated   40/

6. Do you have children? 1 No 2 Yes   41/
If yes, how many? _____ 42-43/
How many live at home? _____ 44-45/

7. What is your present position at MLK? _____ 46-47/
8. What department do you work in at MLK? _____ 48-49/
9. During what year did you start at MLK? _____ 50-51/
10. What other positions have you held at MLK? (If none, skip to
                                                question 11.)

MLK Position		# of months held	
First: _____	52-53/	_____	54-55/
Second: _____	56-57/	_____	58-59/
Third: _____	60-61/	_____	62-63/
Fourth: _____	64-65/	_____	66-67/

11. Were you working before you came to MLK?   1 No   2 Yes   68/
    If yes, what was your previous job? _____ 69-70/
    How long did you have that job? (years)_____ 71-72/
12. What was the main occupation of the head of your household when
    you were a child? _____ 73-74/

GENERAL ATTITUDES ABOUT SOCIETY

	Agree strongly	Agree Moder- ately	Dis- agree Moder- ately	Dis- agree strongly	
13.					
A. The people running this country don't care what happens to people like me.	1	2	3	4	75/
B. People like me don't have any say about what the government does.	1	2	3	4	76/
C. Workers should have a larger role in the management of the place in which they work.	1	2	3	4	77/

14. How would you describe yourself politically?
    1 Conservative   3 Liberal
    2 Moderate   4 Radical   78/

15. What religion were you brought up in?
    1 None   3 Catholic
    2 Protestant   4 Jewish
                                5 Other (specify)
                                   _____   79/

INCOME CATEGORIES

01	$4,000-$5,999	08	$18,000-$19,999
02	$6,000-$7,999	09	$20,000-$21,999
03	$8,000-$9,999	10	$22,000-$23,999
04	$10,000-$11,999	11	$24,000-$25,999
05	$12,000-$13,999	12	$26,000-$27,999
06	$14,000-$15,999	13	$28,000-$29,999
07	$16,000-$17,999	14	$30,000 or over

16. Which category above represents your *own income* from all sources?
Write number of correct category from above here: _____07-08/

17. Which category represents your *total family income* (everyone in
your household).
Write number of category here: _____ 09-10/

18. Which category represents what *you think* your total family income
should be? Write number of category here: _____ 11-12/

ATTACHMENT 2

MLK's DEVELOPMENT—Managerially and Organizationally

INTRODUCTION

As part of the study conducted by the Columbia group this past year, we
would like to get your view of some of the critical events in the devleopment of
MLK since its start. In order to help you remember events we have attempted to
outline a number of phases in the development of MLK. With each phase we
have listed several critical events. We would like to get your views as to whether
these phases make sense to you and whether there are additional critical events
which should be included.

1. HAND RESPONDENT THE LIST OF PHASES AND CRITICAL EVENTS

   a. Have respondent read through it.
   b. Comment on whether the phases make sense—should there be additional
   phases or fewer phases.
2. Ask respondent to go back to the list of phases and events and start with
   Phase I to see if there are any missing important events. If so, write them in.
   This will be repeated for each phase.

Phase One. Incubation. Period of Concept Formulation and Funding

Harold, director Morrisania Ambulatory services, reorganizes specialty services into "clinics" to treat whole person.

Silver proposal rewritten winter of 1965–66 by Wise. Proposal contained essential ideas of Silver's own health teams consisting of nurse, physician, and a family health worker, who was substituted for the social worker.

OEO funds in August 1966.

Three people in community saw proposal (who were they—were there any informal meetings with community people?)

OEO guidelines on community control resulted in strong statement to this effect.

OEO policies influenced, including a training program for nonprofessionals.

Phase Two. Start-up. Period of "Early Enthusiasm and Rapid Achievement"

(Lasts from funding in August 1966 to opening of the Bathgate Center, roughly the first year of operation).

Core group hired. Included Lloyd, Stella, Zahn, Ron Kurahara, Jack Schneider, Ron Brooke, Harriet Bograd.

Survey of community began in August 1966. Purpose was community organizing as well as research.

Apartment meetings began that same month; 150 held.

October 1966 Zahn begins training program in housing project. "Core" training.

December 1966 family health worker training begins; first innovative training.

In March three ad hoc advisory boards formed.

Nurses trained in pediatric care winter and spring (were they trained as practitioners?)

Board elected in late spring.

Bathgate opened in June 1967.

Phase Three: The "Bathgate Period"

(Lasts from opening of Bathgate in June 1967 to opening of Third Avenue Center in 1968).

Training program stymied by problem of upward mobility. Had not broken into college program.

Conflict with advisory board.

Period of role confusion begins.

Strain on charismatic leadership.

Phase Four: Transition

(This period lasts from the move to Third Avenue in 1968 to the Beckhard reform in 1970)

Move from "small to large" increases problem of lack of structure.

Role confusion on health teams.

Lack of defined parameters of health service when health is defined environmentally rather than clinically.

Harold leaves temporarily to travel and find workable plan. (What is date on this?)

Lloyd takes over as acting director in his absence.

Harold goes to Yugoslavia, learns about worker-management.

Harold meets Beckhard.

Phase Five. Beckhard Reconstruction

Harold feels he has found person to begin development of new workable structure. Meetings begin in 1970.

Goals defined with more precision at this time. Discussed by participants. Priorities established. Research is downgraded. Critical decision point about overall mission of the center; Harold wants learning center to train teams. Others opt for delivery model. Latter view prevails.

July 1971 cited as the critical month when major changes are made.

Line and staff functions of physician separated.

Unit manager system initiated.

Beginning of shift to community management.

Health teams trained to be more cooperative and participatory in team interventions.

FHW program taking shape.

Harold leaves

Lloyd becomes director.

Phase Six. Consolidation

(Lasts roughly from 1971 to 1974, the Lloyd-Martin period)

More hard-nosed approach to management.

Weed system initiated.

Emphasis on quality control.

Budget cutbacks.

Cutback in staff.

Emphasis on productivity.

Action-research project of Columbia group initiated; September 1973.

Phase Seven: Community Control

(Present phase)

Ed Martin leaves.

Symbolized by Delores Smith accession to director.

All but one of top and middle managers are "community" people.

Lloyd is now assistant director of medical services.

Action-Research project of Columbia group continues.

Intervention with Beckhard (when?).

Training phasing out.

ATTACHMENT 3

THE DR. MARTIN LUTHER KING, JR. HEALTH CENTER STUDY OF REWARD AND CONTROL PROCEDURES

This questionnaire is being used to obtain data about certain aspects of MLK as an organization. Specifically it focuses on how you and other members of the organization feel about aspects of their jobs and MLK's reward and control procedures. If it is to be useful, it is important that you answer each question frankly and honestly. This is not a test and there are no right or wrong answers.

This study is being carried out by a research group from the Columbia University Graduate School of Business under the direction of Dr. Noel Tichy, Associate Professor of Business, Columbia University.

The answers to the questions in this questionnaire will be processed by computers and summarized in statistical form so that your responses will remain confidential. No one in this organization will have access to any information about any individual employee or to any individual employee's answers on this questionnaire. All individual questionnaires will be returned to Columbia University and will remain there under the confidential safeguard of the University.

The results of this study are intended to help improve the reward and control procedures at MLK. The results of the study will be shared with all those who participate in filling out the questionnaire in such a way as to protect individual confidentiality. In addition, a committee made up of management and professional supervisors will be provided with feedback in such a form as to protect all individuals' confidentiality. This committee will work with the research group to explore the implications of the research for changes in MLK's reward and control procedures.

Thank you in advance for your cooperation. We hope that you will find this questionnaire interesting and thought provoking.

GENERAL INSTRUCTIONS

Most of the questions in this survey ask that you check one of several numbers that appear on a scale to the right of the question. You should choose the one number that best matches the description of how you feel about the question or statement. For example, if you were asked how much you agree with the statement "I like the Bronx" and you felt that you strongly agreed, you would check the number under "strongly agree" as so:

How much do you agree or disagree with the following statement?	strongly disagree	disagree	slightly disagree	neither agree nor disagree	slightly agree	agree	strongly agree
a. I like the Bronx.	(1)	(2)	(3)	(4)	(5)	(6)	(7)

Please note that the numbered responses may mean different things for different parts of the questionnaire. Therefore, be sure to read the instructions that appear in the boxes and be sure to read the headings over the numbers before you check your answers.

Study identification number:_____	761	1:01-03
(do not fill in)		1:04-06
Your job title: (check one) (1) nurse		1:07
(2) dentist		
(3) family health worker		
(4) physician		
(5) medical assistant		
(6) dental assistant	999	1:08-10

1. DIFFERENT PEOPLE WANT
DIFFERENT THINGS FROM
THEIR JOBS. BELOW IS A
LIST OF DIFFERENT ASPECTS
OF A JOB. HOW IMPORTANT
ARE EACH OF THE FOLLOWING
TO YOU?

HOW IMPORTANT IS . . .

	moderately important or less		quite important			extremely important		
a. the friendliness of the people you work with.	(1)	(2)	(3)	(4)	(5)	(6)	(7)	1:11
b. the amount of freedom you have on your job.	(1)	(2)	(3)	(4)	(5)	(6)	(7)	1:12
c. the chances you have to be exposed to new clinical cases.	(1)	(2)	(3)	(4)	(5)	(6)	(7)	1:13
d. the opportunity to be intellectually stimulated.	(1)	(2)	(3)	(4)	(5)	(6)	(7)	1:14
e. the respect you receive from the people you work with.	(1)	(2)	(3)	(4)	(5)	(6)	(7)	1:15
f. the chances you have to accomplish something worthwhile.	(1)	(2)	(3)	(4)	(5)	(6)	(7)	1:16

HOW IMPORTANT IS . . .

g. the amount of pay you get.	(1)	(2)	(3)	(4)	(5)	(6)	(7)	1:17
h. the chances you have to do things you do best.	(1)	(2)	(3)	(4)	(5)	(6)	(7)	1:18
i. the chances you have to do something that makes you feel good about yourself as a person.	(1)	(2)	(3)	(4)	(5)	(6)	(7)	1:19
j. the way you are treated by the people you work with.	(1)	(2)	(3)	(4)	(5)	(6)	(7)	1:20
k. your chances for getting ahead in this organization.	(1)	(2)	(3)	(4)	(5)	(6)	(7)	1:21

HOW IMPORTANT IS . . .

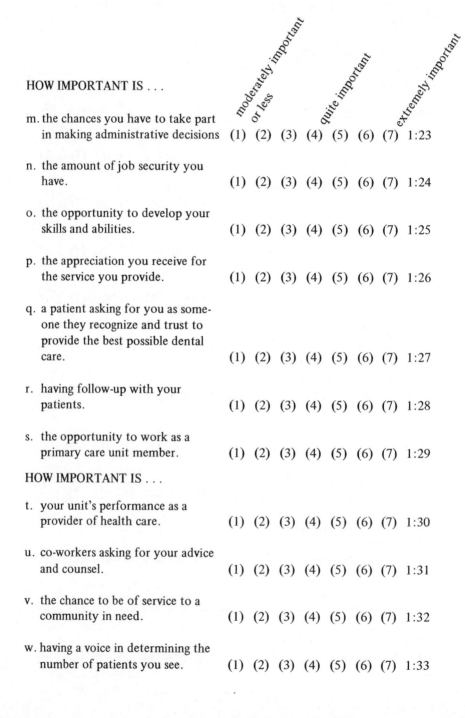

m. the chances you have to take part
   in making administrative decisions   (1) (2) (3) (4) (5) (6) (7) 1:23

n. the amount of job security you
   have.   (1) (2) (3) (4) (5) (6) (7) 1:24

o. the opportunity to develop your
   skills and abilities.   (1) (2) (3) (4) (5) (6) (7) 1:25

p. the appreciation you receive for
   the service you provide.   (1) (2) (3) (4) (5) (6) (7) 1:26

q. a patient asking for you as some-
   one they recognize and trust to
   provide the best possible dental
   care.   (1) (2) (3) (4) (5) (6) (7) 1:27

r. having follow-up with your
   patients.   (1) (2) (3) (4) (5) (6) (7) 1:28

s. the opportunity to work as a
   primary care unit member.   (1) (2) (3) (4) (5) (6) (7) 1:29

HOW IMPORTANT IS . . .

t. your unit's performance as a
   provider of health care.   (1) (2) (3) (4) (5) (6) (7) 1:30

u. co-workers asking for your advice
   and counsel.   (1) (2) (3) (4) (5) (6) (7) 1:31

v. the chance to be of service to a
   community in need.   (1) (2) (3) (4) (5) (6) (7) 1:32

w. having a voice in determining the
   number of patients you see.   (1) (2) (3) (4) (5) (6) (7) 1:33

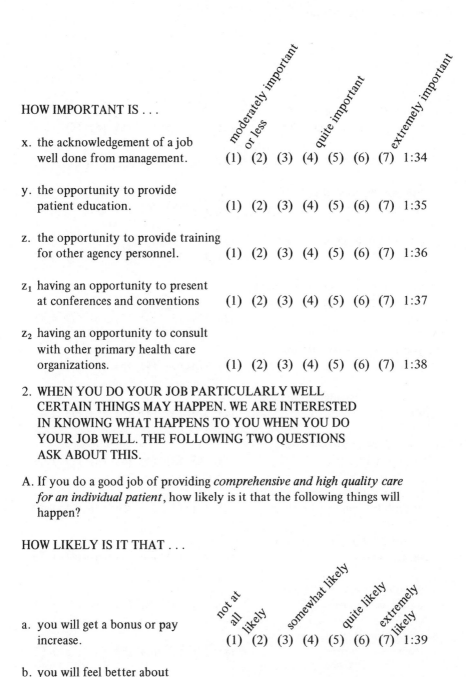

HOW IMPORTANT IS . . .

moderately important or less *quite important* *extremely important*

x. the acknowledgement of a job
   well done from management.   (1) (2) (3) (4) (5) (6) (7) 1:34

y. the opportunity to provide
   patient education.   (1) (2) (3) (4) (5) (6) (7) 1:35

z. the opportunity to provide training
   for other agency personnel.   (1) (2) (3) (4) (5) (6) (7) 1:36

z_1 having an opportunity to present
   at conferences and conventions   (1) (2) (3) (4) (5) (6) (7) 1:37

z_2 having an opportunity to consult
   with other primary health care
   organizations.   (1) (2) (3) (4) (5) (6) (7) 1:38

2. WHEN YOU DO YOUR JOB PARTICULARLY WELL
   CERTAIN THINGS MAY HAPPEN. WE ARE INTERESTED
   IN KNOWING WHAT HAPPENS TO YOU WHEN YOU DO
   YOUR JOB WELL. THE FOLLOWING TWO QUESTIONS
   ASK ABOUT THIS.

A. If you do a good job of providing *comprehensive and high quality care
   for an individual patient*, how likely is it that the following things will
   happen?

HOW LIKELY IS IT THAT . . .

not at all likely *somewhat likely* *quite likely* *extremely likely*

a. you will get a bonus or pay
   increase.   (1) (2) (3) (4) (5) (6) (7) 1:39

b. you will feel better about
   yourself as a person.   (1) (2) (3) (4) (5) (6) (7) 1:40

HOW LIKELY IS IT THAT . . .

	not at all likely		somewhat likely		quite likely		extremely likely	
c. you will have an opportunity to develop your skills and abilities.	(1)	(2)	(3)	(4)	(5)	(6)	(7)	1:41
d. you will have better job security.	(1)	(2)	(3)	(4)	(5)	(6)	(7)	1:42
e. you will be given chances to learn new things.	(1)	(2)	(3)	(4)	(5)	(6)	(7)	1:43
f. you will be promoted or get a better job.	(1)	(2)	(3)	(4)	(5)	(6)	(7)	1:44
g. you will get a feeling that you've accomplished something worthwhile.	(1)	(2)	(3)	(4)	(5)	(6)	(7)	1:45
h. you will have more freedom on your job.	(1)	(2)	(3)	(4)	(5)	(6)	(7)	1:46
i. you will be stimulated intellectually	(1)	(2)	(3)	(4)	(5)	(6)	(7)	1:47
j. you will be appreciated by your patients.	(1)	(2)	(3)	(4)	(5)	(6)	(7)	1:48
k. your patients will recognize you and ask for you to treat them.	(1)	(2)	(3)	(4)	(5)	(6)	(7)	1:49
l. your team's performance will be a good one.	(1)	(2)	(3)	(4)	(5)	(6)	(7)	1:50
m. co-workers will ask you for advice and counsel.	(1)	(2)	(3)	(4)	(5)	(6)	(7)	1:51
n. you will feel you have provided quality health care.	(1)	(2)	(3)	(4)	(5)	(6)	(7)	1:52
o. your co-workers will treat you better.	(1)	(2)	(3)	(4)	(5)	(6)	(7)	1:53

HOW LIKELY IS IT THAT . . .

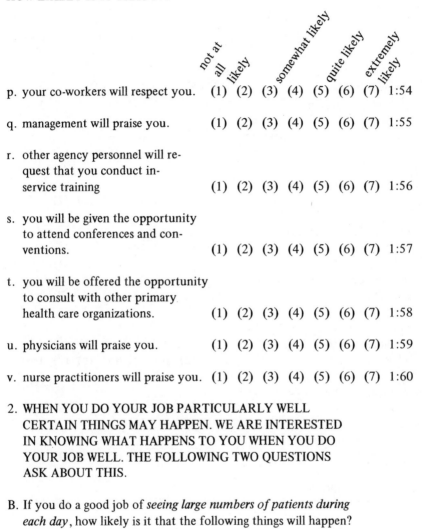

p. your co-workers will respect you.   (1) (2) (3) (4) (5) (6) (7) 1:54

q. management will praise you.   (1) (2) (3) (4) (5) (6) (7) 1:55

r. other agency personnel will request that you conduct in-
   service training   (1) (2) (3) (4) (5) (6) (7) 1:56

s. you will be given the opportunity
   to attend conferences and con-
   ventions.   (1) (2) (3) (4) (5) (6) (7) 1:57

t. you will be offered the opportunity
   to consult with other primary
   health care organizations.   (1) (2) (3) (4) (5) (6) (7) 1:58

u. physicians will praise you.   (1) (2) (3) (4) (5) (6) (7) 1:59

v. nurse practitioners will praise you. (1) (2) (3) (4) (5) (6) (7) 1:60

2. WHEN YOU DO YOUR JOB PARTICULARLY WELL
   CERTAIN THINGS MAY HAPPEN. WE ARE INTERESTED
   IN KNOWING WHAT HAPPENS TO YOU WHEN YOU DO
   YOUR JOB WELL. THE FOLLOWING TWO QUESTIONS
   ASK ABOUT THIS.

B. If you do a good job of *seeing large numbers of patients during
   each day*, how likely is it that the following things will happen?

HOW LIKELY IS IT THAT . . .

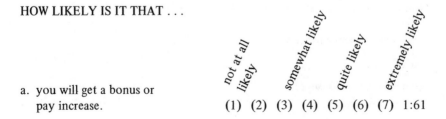

a. you will get a bonus or
   pay increase.   (1) (2) (3) (4) (5) (6) (7) 1:61

HOW LIKELY IS IT THAT . . .

		not at all likely	likely	somewhat likely		quite likely		extremely likely	
b.	you will feel better about yourself as a person.	(1)	(2)	(3)	(4)	(5)	(6)	(7)	1:62
c.	you will have an opportunity to develop your skills and abilities.	(1)	(2)	(3)	(4)	(5)	(6)	(7)	1:63
d.	you will have better job security.	(1)	(2)	(3)	(4)	(5)	(6)	(7)	1:64
e.	you will be given chances to learn new things.	(1)	(2)	(3)	(4)	(5)	(6)	(7)	1:65
f.	you will be promoted or get a better job.	(1)	(2)	(3)	(4)	(5)	(6)	(7)	1:66
g.	you will get a feeling that you've accomplished something worthwhile.	(1)	(2)	(3)	(4)	(5)	(6)	(7)	1:67
h.	you will have more freedom on your job.	(1)	(2)	(3)	(4)	(5)	(6)	(7)	1:68
i.	you will be stimulated intellectually.	(1)	(2)	(3)	(4)	(5)	(6)	(7)	1:69
j.	you will be appreciated by your patients.	(1)	(2)	(3)	(4)	(5)	(6)	(7)	1:70
k.	your patients will recognize you and ask for you to treat them.	(1)	(2)	(3)	(4)	(5)	(6)	(7)	1:71
l.	your team's performance will be a good one.	(1)	(2)	(3)	(4)	(5)	(6)	(7)	1:72
m.	co-workers will ask you for advice and counsel.	(1)	(2)	(3)	(4)	(5)	(6)	(7)	1:73

HOW LIKELY IS IT THAT . . .

not at all likely   *likely*   *somewhat likely*   *quite likely*   *extremely likely*

n. you will feel you have provided
   quality health care.   (1) (2) (3) (4) (5) (6) (7) 1:74

o. your co-workers will treat you
   better.   (1) (2) (3) (4) (5) (6) (7) 1:75

p. your co-workers will respect you.   (1) (2) (3) (4) (5) (6) (7) 1:76

q. management will praise you.   (1) (2) (3) (4) (5) (6) (7) 1:77

r. other agency personnel will request that you conduct in-
   service training   (1) (2) (3) (4) (5) (6) (7) 1:78

s. you will be given the opportunity
   to attend conferences and con-
   ventions.   (1) (2) (3) (4) (5) (6) (7) 1:79

t. you will be offered the opportunity
   to consult with other primary
   health care organizations   (1) (2) (3) (4) (5) (6) (7) 1:80

u. physicians will praise you.   (1) (2) (3) (4) (5) (6) (7) 2:11

v. nurse practitioners will praise you.   (1) (2) (3) (4) (5) (6) (7) 2:12

3. IN THE QUESTION YOU ANSWERED BEFORE, YOU
   RATED THE IMPORTANT ASPECTS OF YOUR WORK.

   HERE YOU ARE BEING ASKED SOMETHING
   DIFFERENT. IN THIS QUESTION, PLEASE
   INDICATE *HOW SATISFIED YOU ARE* WITH
   EACH OF THE FOLLOWING ASPECTS OF YOUR
   JOB.

HOW SATISFIED ARE YOU WITH . . .

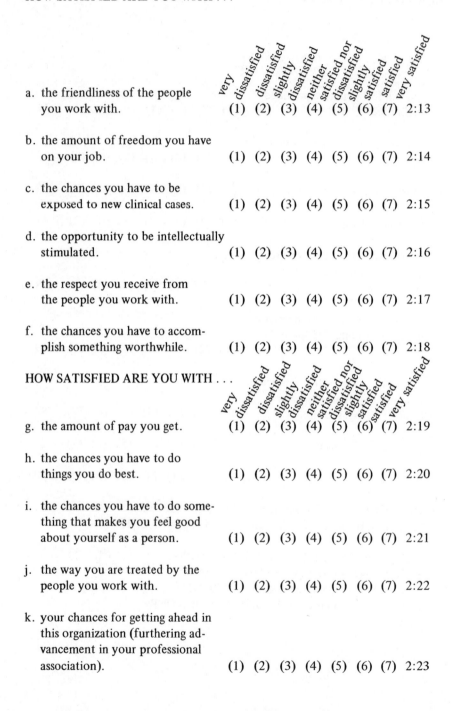

a. the friendliness of the people
   you work with.   (1) (2) (3) (4) (5) (6) (7) 2:13

b. the amount of freedom you have
   on your job.   (1) (2) (3) (4) (5) (6) (7) 2:14

c. the chances you have to be
   exposed to new clinical cases.   (1) (2) (3) (4) (5) (6) (7) 2:15

d. the opportunity to be intellectually
   stimulated.   (1) (2) (3) (4) (5) (6) (7) 2:16

e. the respect you receive from
   the people you work with.   (1) (2) (3) (4) (5) (6) (7) 2:17

f. the chances you have to accom-
   plish something worthwhile.   (1) (2) (3) (4) (5) (6) (7) 2:18

HOW SATISFIED ARE YOU WITH . . .

g. the amount of pay you get.   (1) (2) (3) (4) (5) (6) (7) 2:19

h. the chances you have to do
   things you do best.   (1) (2) (3) (4) (5) (6) (7) 2:20

i. the chances you have to do something that makes you feel good
   about yourself as a person.   (1) (2) (3) (4) (5) (6) (7) 2:21

j. the way you are treated by the
   people you work with.   (1) (2) (3) (4) (5) (6) (7) 2:22

k. your chances for getting ahead in
   this organization (furthering ad-
   vancement in your professional
   association).   (1) (2) (3) (4) (5) (6) (7) 2:23

HOW SATISFIED ARE YOU WITH . . .

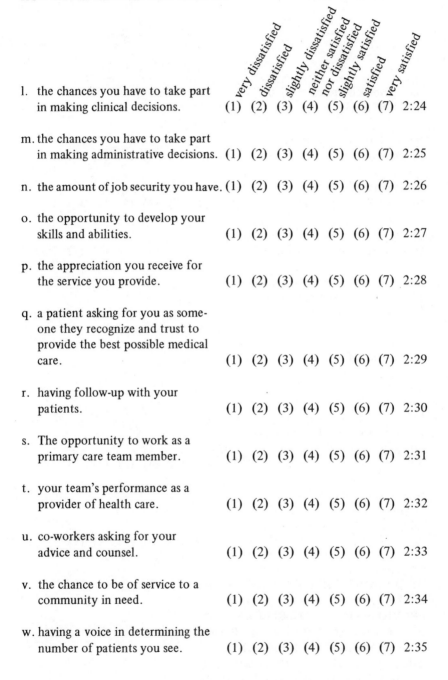

l. the chances you have to take part
in making clinical decisions.   (1) (2) (3) (4) (5) (6) (7) 2:24

m. the chances you have to take part
in making administrative decisions. (1) (2) (3) (4) (5) (6) (7) 2:25

n. the amount of job security you have. (1) (2) (3) (4) (5) (6) (7) 2:26

o. the opportunity to develop your
skills and abilities.   (1) (2) (3) (4) (5) (6) (7) 2:27

p. the appreciation you receive for
the service you provide.   (1) (2) (3) (4) (5) (6) (7) 2:28

q. a patient asking for you as some-
one they recognize and trust to
provide the best possible medical
care.   (1) (2) (3) (4) (5) (6) (7) 2:29

r. having follow-up with your
patients.   (1) (2) (3) (4) (5) (6) (7) 2:30

s. The opportunity to work as a
primary care team member.   (1) (2) (3) (4) (5) (6) (7) 2:31

t. your team's performance as a
provider of health care.   (1) (2) (3) (4) (5) (6) (7) 2:32

u. co-workers asking for your
advice and counsel.   (1) (2) (3) (4) (5) (6) (7) 2:33

v. the chance to be of service to a
community in need.   (1) (2) (3) (4) (5) (6) (7) 2:34

w. having a voice in determining the
number of patients you see.   (1) (2) (3) (4) (5) (6) (7) 2:35

HOW SATISFIED ARE YOU WITH . . .

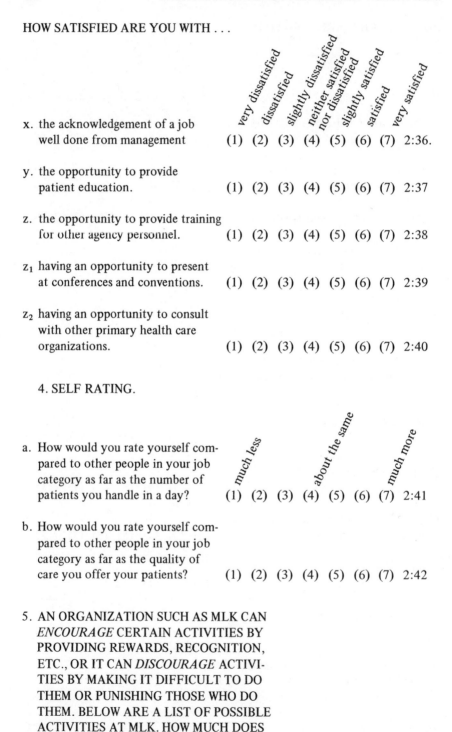

x. the acknowledgement of a job
   well done from management   (1)   (2)   (3)   (4)   (5)   (6)   (7)   2:36.

y. the opportunity to provide
   patient education.   (1)   (2)   (3)   (4)   (5)   (6)   (7)   2:37

z. the opportunity to provide training
   for other agency personnel.   (1)   (2)   (3)   (4)   (5)   (6)   (7)   2:38

z_1 having an opportunity to present
   at conferences and conventions.   (1)   (2)   (3)   (4)   (5)   (6)   (7)   2:39

z_2 having an opportunity to consult
   with other primary health care
   organizations.   (1)   (2)   (3)   (4)   (5)   (6)   (7)   2:40

4. SELF RATING.

a. How would you rate yourself compared to other people in your job
   category as far as the number of
   patients you handle in a day?   (1)   (2)   (3)   (4)   (5)   (6)   (7)   2:41

b. How would you rate yourself compared to other people in your job
   category as far as the quality of
   care you offer your patients?   (1)   (2)   (3)   (4)   (5)   (6)   (7)   2:42

5. AN ORGANIZATION SUCH AS MLK CAN
   ENCOURAGE CERTAIN ACTIVITIES BY
   PROVIDING REWARDS, RECOGNITION,
   ETC., OR IT CAN *DISCOURAGE* ACTIVI-
   TIES BY MAKING IT DIFFICULT TO DO
   THEM OR PUNISHING THOSE WHO DO
   THEM. BELOW ARE A LIST OF POSSIBLE
   ACTIVITIES AT MLK. HOW MUCH DOES
   THE MANAGEMENT OF MLK ENCOURAGE
   OR DISCOURAGE EACH?:

a. improving existing medical
   protocols and procedures.   (1) (2) (3) (4) (5) (6) (7) 2:43

b. spending time on patient
   education.   (1) (2) (3) (4) (5) (6) (7) 2:44

c. seeing large numbers of patients. (1) (2) (3) (4) (5) (6) (7) 2:45

d. developing new programs and/or
   ideas to improve patient
   education.   (1) (2) (3) (4) (5) (6) (7) 2:46

e. providing training and development
   for other staff (conducting in-
   service training, etc.)   (1) (2) (3) (4) (5) (6) (7) 2:47

f. providing high-quality care.   (1) (2) (3) (4) (5) (6) (7) 2:48

g. doing activities which help make
   the team more effective.   (1) (2) (3) (4) (5) (6) (7) 2:49

h. acquiring new knowledge and skills
   related to your job.   (1) (2) (3) (4) (5) (6) (7) 2:50

6. FINALLY, WE ARE INTERESTED IN WHAT HAPPENS
   AT MLK WHEN YOU DO NOT SEE MANY PATIENTS
   AND WHEN THE QUALITY OF CARE IS NOT GOOD.

   PLEASE WRITE BELOW WHAT HAPPENS WHEN . . .

a. You (or other at MLK) do not see the expected
   number of patients:

   _____

_____

_____

_____

b. You (or others at MLK) provide poor quality care: _____

_____

_____

_____

_____

	1968	1970	1972	1974	1976
Patient information					
Residents in area served	45,000	45,000	90,000*	90,000 (est.)	71,000 (est.)
Percent Black		74	62	54	47*
Percent Puerto Rican		23	36	41	45
Individuals registered and receiving care in past 18 months		26,800	39,000	43,300	39,000
Individuals registered per team (average)		1,500	4,600	5,000	3,500
Patient services					
Visits to health center		153,000	182,000	188,000	167,400
Health care units		81,000	84,000	93,000	87,000
Emergency room		31,000	49,000	44,000	40,000
Specialty unit		n.a.	27,000	27,000	22,000
Dental unit		n.a.	22,000	24,000	18,000
Home visits, FHW's		68,000	40,000	25,000	12,000
Pharmacy prescriptions		154,000	221,000	257,000	250,000
Average number of visits per registered individual		5.7	4.7	4.3	4.3
Staff (full-time equivalents)					
Total employees	419	583	432	381	360
Health services	280	305	329	300	245
Administration	139	278	103	81	115
Typical health care teams (8)					
Family health workers	6	6	6	6	4
Public health nurse	2	2.5	2	2	1.5
Pediatricians	1	1	1	1	1
Internists	1	1	2	2	1.5
Secretaries	1	1	1	1	1.6
Dentists	1	1	1	1	.5
Typical unit (serves two teams)					
Medical assistants	5	4	7	7	6
Receptionists	3	3	3	3	3
Unit manager	1	1	1	1	1

Budgeted Statements of Operations
1968-76

	1968	1970	1974	1976
Patient Service Revenues				
Medicaid	$ 577,500		$3,800,000	$3,900,000
		$1,509,000		
Medicare			70,000	100,000
	15,000			
Self-pay and other third party			30,000	127,000
Total Revenues:	$4,195,615	$6,112,168	$8,600,000	$7,161,000
Expenses				
Total personnel expenses (salary and fringes)	$2,688,513	$5,221,744	$6,138,826	$6,519,438
Other operating expenses	2,778,290	2,050,622	1,070,088	856,972
	$5,466,803	$7,272,366	$7,208,914	$7,376,410
	($1,271,188)	($1,160,198)	($1,391,085)	($ 215,410)

*Catchment area of the center extended from two city health areas to five. Census figures for these areas are estimated for 1974, 1976.

Source: Compiled by Kathleen Dalton. These figures were reported to us by Delores Smith, director, and are not taken from actual accounting records.

THE PROBLEM-ORIENTED RECORD
Jeanne M. Reed, RRA

Hospitals and health centers all over the country are interested in, or in the process of, converting from the traditional system of record-keeping to a new method: the problem-oriented record. Rather than being a collection of fragmented, unstructured bits of information, the problem-oriented method encourages production of a logical and complete document relating to the patient's problems. A problem list serves as the table of contents or index to the rest of the information contained within the record.

This relatively new concept was developed by Dr. Lawrence Weed, who has initiated the system through teaching, training and lecturing. Physicians who have followed this approach have been instrumental in introducing it into their own office practice or hospital. The problem-oriented medical record consists of four elements: 1) data base, 2) problem list, 3) initial plan, and 4) progress notes. It requires the physician to become disciplined in the collection and orderly recording of information.

The Data Base

The data base represents all the information collected through history-taking, physical examination, and reports of laboratory tests and x-ray procedures. Emphasis is placed on the patient profile, which is an expansion of the traditional social history and the statement of present illness, so that the physician may have an indepth understanding of his patient and the many variables that affect his state of health. By describing the problems and the history separately, the statement of illness will include a description of symptoms, objective data, significant negative findings, and pertinent information concerning previous treatment.

The Problem List

The problem list is compiled from pertinent information found in the data base, each problem being listed by number. The problem may be of a social, medical or psychiatric nature, supported by the data in the record, and it may be a diagnosis, symptom or unusual physiologic finding. Traditional medicine usually upheld the concept of stating only the diagnosis and treating the patient for the disease he might have. The problem-oriented system permits dissemination of more organized knowledge by analyzing symptoms, physiological findings and abnormal test results as well as diagnoses. By outlining the foregoing in an easily read, structured format, the practitioner can analyze the aggregated problems and come to a more complete diagnosis.

The problem list is of such importance to the practitioner that it should be kept on the front of the record and must be kept current. This will aid anyone viewing the patient's record in obtaining a longitudinal picture of his health status. Problems should be entered on the list as soon as the data base is compiled. Because of the ongoing nature of this list, new problems are added, and treated problems are kept on the list and annotated with statements indicating resolution.

The Initial Plan

The initial plan is related to each problem on the list and includes the proposed management of each problem along with possible diagnosis. This documented evidence helps to correlate the problem and its management with other problems. The plan should be written to include patient education.

The Progress Note

The progress note is also problem-oriented. It is written by the physician or any practitioner caring for the patient. Each problem in the record is delineated and numbered, thus making it easy to relate back to the original problem list.

The progress note is divided into: subjective data, objective data, assessment (interpretation) and plan, which is commonly referred to as SOAP. By using this structural method for each problem, anyone can see at a glance what the physician has in mind for dealing with each problem.

Flow sheets can be used in the record to supplement the continuation sheets. The physician selects the parameters to be measured, such as the recording of vital signs, physical findings, lab data, input/output, medications, depending on the needs of the patient. The flow sheet, with all the above data, serves to alert the physician to changes which could have significant bearing on the illness or management of the patient.

Summary

Advocates of the problem-oriented system of record-keeping feel that it is a vast improvement if used wisely. While it may take time to introduce and implement the system, it has many advantages. First, each problem can be treated in relation to other problems. Second, the important facts are readily available so that problems can be evaluated and current status, previous findings and treatment can be assessed. Third, the table of contents, provided by the problem list, permits any physician to follow any problem in the the progress notes. Finally, the system encourages a better relationship between an attending physician and an intern or resident because each can more readily understand the other's methods and plans by reading the chart entries. Family care benefits from the problem-oriented method because a link can be established between a family problem list and the individual problem lists, thus furnishing a composite picture of the family as a whole.

THE MEDICAL CARE EVALUATION COMMITTEE
Jeanne M. Reed, RRA

The Medical Care Evaluation committee held its first meeting on February 15, 1971. The Committee was established to evaluate the care of families and make recommendations to practitioners for improving the quality of care. It was not the intent of the Committee to police the activities of practitioners.

The members were the Medical Director, a senior internist, a pediatrician, an obstetrician, a nurse, a licensed practitioner nurse supervisor, a Community Health Advocacy representative, a family health worker and a dentist. It was hoped that a representative of the Community Advisory Board would also sit on the Committee, but it was not possible to arrange this during working hours. Strict confidentiality concerning Committee meetings and actions was enforced, and it was made clear that any breach of the confidentiality could serve as a basis for dismissal from the Committee.

The group met once a week for two hours to evaluate medical care based on input from three sources:
  I.   Chart Review (see page 191).
  II. Outcome Review
       a. Deaths within the community
       b. Drug reactions in the Center
       c. Hospital admissions referred from the Center or registered patients admitted to a hospital
  III. Patient grievance and patient satisfaction.

As the Committee progressed, it realized that a form was needed in order to perform chart review. The first form was used on March 30, 1971, when actual chart review began and has been revised several times.

From The Dr. Martin Luther King, Jr. Health Center, Sixth Annual Report, 1973.

About four months after its inception, the Committee decided to retain the original permanent membership. Over the years, however, the membership has had some additions and changes, such as a representative from the Office of Professional Affairs serving as secretary to the group and the resignation of the licensed practical nurse supervisor. I became a Committee member because I had been working on the Chart Review Committee, which was an early attempt to establish criteria for review of charts. Also, as a medical record administrator I had a particular interest in chart audit.

To increase our knowledge of auditing systems the Committee has studied pertinent articles and invited experts to discuss audit with us.

I. Chart Review

A typical Committee meeting began with chart review. Each week a different member presented a chart which had been reviewed by him, using the medical care evaluation form. Copies of the completed form were distributed to the group. After the Committee suggested additional recommendations, the reviewer had the responsibility for presenting them to the appropriate team. Comments from the meeting with the team were presented at the next meeting and follow-up measures were instituted two months after the initial presentation to insure proper care. A team member was invited to attend the meeting each week provided that his team was not being reviewed.

II. Outcome Review

Deaths

Input of information on deaths of patients came through three channels.

1. the MLK attending physician in the hospital;
2. team members who provided care to the patient; and
3. a review of a mortality list of MLK patients obtained from the Department of Health.

All material collected was discussed by the Committee to determine whether care given by the Center was inadequate and possibly contributed to the death. Then recommendations pertaining to future prevention of similar circumstances were made. These included:

1. improved care of acute incidents;
2. stricter protocols for care of patients with chronic disease; and
3. means for preventing accidents.

Drug Reactions

The Office of Professional Affairs and Operations Analysis Department collected data regarding drug reactions from various sources, such as team members, emergency room physicians, and hospitals. This information was presented to the Committee when appropriate. The Committee then made recommendations pertaining to the future prevention of similar occurrences such as:

1. use of a drug profile;
2. improvement in accessibility of a medical record when treating a patient in the emergency room; and
3. stamping outside of the medical record to indicate drug sensitivity.

These recommendations were sent to the Director of Health Services for follow-up.

Hospital Admissions

Unusual circumstances of hospital admissions were discussed. Examples of these were:

1. medical and obstetrical complications;
2. patient complaints; and
3. accidents occurring during hospitalization.

Attempts were made to resolve the problems and prevent further occurrences.

III. Patient Grievance

A member from the Community Health Advocacy Department was responsible for handling patient grievances. (See Patient Grievance Report, page 220). Major complaints of patients, such as breach of confidentiality, rudeness on the part of the staff and a sense of mistreatment as expressed by the patient or the family, were addressed to the Committee for further correction. The Committee either made recommendations for further action or informed the CHA representative that his approach was acceptable.

The representative from CHA was also called upon to submit a consumer-satisfaction form for the family whose care was being audited by the chart review. This form indicated both the awareness of the family regarding availability of services and their comments on the quality of these services. If the family commented unfavorably, appropriate measures were taken to correct the situation whether it was an individual or a Center-wide problem.

In the last few months the Committee has "shifted gears" from standard evaluation procedures as listed above to aiding the teams in developing protocols and establishing means for cross-team evaluation. The purpose of the change is to obtain greater involvement of members of the team.

MEDICAL CARE EVALUATION—CHART REVIEW*

Reviewer: _____   Internist: _____

Name: _____   Pediatrician:_____

Address & Team: _____   PHN: _____

Registration Date:_____   FHW: _____

FAMILY TREE   MAJOR FAMILY & INDIVIDUAL
                                                        PROBLEMS
                                                          1.
                                                          2.
                                                          3.
                                                          4.
                                                          5.
                                                          6.
                                                          7.
                                                          8.
                                                          9.
                                                         10.

                                      CHECK LIST (X=Means Adequate)
                                                        (O=Means Inadequate)

1. TEAM FUNCTION
    A)   Communication—Problems communicated with appropriate member
    B)   Coordination of problems and implementation
    C)   Follow-up

2. FAMILY FOLDER
    A)   Family Structure
          Living Quarters
          Economics
          List of Medical & Social Problems

*Actual form is four pages.

Problem Sheet on Family Folder

Plan & Follow-up

B)   Summary of Family Folder: yearly (Routine) 6 months (Problem Family)

C)   Problem Oriented Notes (Weed) with follow-up

D)   Summary of Team Conference with follow-up

3. FAMILY CARE AUDIT

PEDIATRICS

1. Subjective: Chief complaint

   Interval History and past history

2. Objective: Physical, including growth chart and lab. data

3. Interpretation & Plan: Impression & follow-up including:

   Health Supervision

   Standard procedure

   Consultation & treatment plan

4. Format: Problem oriented notes with problem oriented list

OBSTETRICS & GYNECOLOGY

I. 1. Subjective: History

   2. Objective: Physical including lab data

   3. Interpretation & Plan plus follow-thru: use of problem sheet

   4. Legibility and completeness of records

II. Above format a satisfactory base-line to apply to:

Prenatal Care

Postpartum Care

Family Planning

Papaniolau smear screening

Gynecological problems

INTERNAL MEDICINE

1. History and physical examination

2. Lab: CBC, Urine, Serology, Sickle Cell Prep, BUN, Choc, PPBS, Tine Test, Chest X-ray

3. Problem identification and follow-thru—use of problem sheet

4. Legibility

DENTAL DEPARTMENT

1. Preventive Dentistry

2. Formal Treatment Plan

3. Complete Pre-treatment records

   A)   Medical History

   B)   X-ray

    C)   Release Authorization Form
    D)   Continuation Sheet
4. Completeness of Treatment
    A)   In-Progress
    B)   Recall
    C)   Complete

FAMILY HEALTH WORKER CHART REVIEW
Paula Lamot, Senior Family Health Worker

To assure that each patient of the Health Center receives high-quality care and follow-up, family charts are reviewed periodically. Originally, the public health nurse was responsible for chart review every six months, but as the family health worker gained knowledge of both the medical and social field, he or she became responsible for chart review once a year.

The family health worker uses the Family and Individual Plan (see page 195) for chart review. The plan is divided into four areas (doctor, public health nurse, family health worker and referrals), and the name of each member of the household appears on the sheet along with the practitioner who saw him or her.

The objectives of the chart review are to:

1) maintain good health care follow-up;
2) make sure that patients get basic health-maintenance care;
3) arrange for follow-up appointsments on abnormal lab tests;
4) assess health care when patients are referred outside the team;
5) check social assessments; and
6) make every team member aware of whether a patient has been using the Center.

The chart is also reviewed to be sure that all the necessary forms are included and complete, that all problems entered on the problem list form are either treated or adequately accounted for, and that no fragments of other patients' records are misplaced in the chart reviewed.

Areas that require further consideration are listed under the appropriate professions in the Family and Individual Plan. Appointments are then made with the patient needing more care. The chart review is kept in the family folder so that the practitioner can evaluate and follow through on the recommendations of the family health worker.

Most of the time team members have demonstrated adequate health care, and they have accepted constructive criticism from the Medical Care Evaluation Committee. Through auditing the charts, team members have been able to improve the quality of patient care. Out of the recognition of the need for ongoing evaluation of our practices the following systems have been started:

Chart Review

Ongoing and systematic chart review of all nurse practitioners by the Nursing Professional Supervisor.

Protocols

Awareness of the need for protocols arose simultaneously in all professional groups at MLK. They provide solid guidelines for practice and chart review. There are protocols for care in pediatrics, obstetrics and gynecology and the new focus area of adult primary medicine.

Committees of nurses have formed or reactivated to establish (with physician consultation) criteria in the forms of protocols for primary care. The committees now functioning are:

Pediatrics: protocols are already in use for health maintenance, strept throat infections, urinary tract infection, anemia, acute gastroenteritis, pneumonia, asthma, otitis media, high blood lead levels, convulsive disorders.

Venereal disease: protocols are established for the management of gonorrhea and syphilis all by team members. (See VD report, page 215).

Obstetrics and Gynecology: prenatal, home visit, and office postpartum protocols are already in use and gynecology protocols are being developed.

Adult Care: This committee has just been formed.

Internists and pediatricians are working in their own groups on protocols as well, which nurses will approve and use as indicated. One of the critical factors is for all groups to agree on the minimum standards of good care.

Our current work is aimed at implementing, as soon as possible, a thorough and ongoing review of nurse practice at MLK, based on solid criteria known to all and accepted as good health care by nurses and physicians at this Center. In addition, we hope to improve the supervisory relationship of Health Center physicians with team nurses in all areas for our patients' good and our mutual satety in practice. Finally, as we develop more protocols in the area of adult care, we will begin to open that field more and more to our nurse practitioners and fill an important need of our teams.

PEDIATRIC ASSESSMENT   Gita Mukerjee, M.D.

The pediatricians at the King Health Center have been a very active and aggressive group in both improving the quality of their practice and teaching nurses and paramedical personnel.

The first chart review in the Center was done through the Medical Care Evaluation Committee. Forms were devised for an objective appraisal of family records. The Chief of Pediatrics, who reviewed individual pediatric charts weekly, felt that a more in-depth evaluation was needed for pediatric care. She maintained that if protocols of both health maintenance and chronic disease maintenance were devised, the quality of care could be more objectively evaluated. She presented this idea to the pediatricians. They unanimously agreed to the need for the development of standard protocols and a chart evaluation format.

Protocols

The purpose of protocols is to define prescribed approaches to common illness so that the care of patients will be uniform. It also will provide guidelines to nurses and family health workers.

The pediatricians decided to use the problem-oriented format of subjective, objective, assessment and plan (SOAP) as the format for the protocols. Nine common illnesses were selected. These are 1) urinary tract infections, 2) acute gastroenteritis, 3) anemia, 4) pneumonia, 5) asthma, 6) otitis media, 7) high blood lead levels, 8) convulsive disorders, and 9) strept throat. Each pediatrician researched and established a protocol for one of the above illnesses. A committee, chaired by a resident in social pediatrics, was appointed to review the submitted formats. The result was a concise compilation of standardized care for nine common illnesses.

Chart Evaluation (See pages 200–201).

The purpose of the chart evaluation is to assess the physicians' performances in relation to predetermined criteria. The format is divided into three areas: 1) non-negotiable checklist, 2) history and management checklist, and 3) the reviewers subjective assessment of the quality of care.

Non-negotiable Checklist

In the context of medical care, "non-negotiable" implies that certain items must be included in the examination. This means that in the course of a physical examination pediatricians must include items such as hematocrit, sickle cell prep and tine test. The pedicatricians determined these criteria and established a health maintenance protocol for immunizations.

History and Management Checklist

This area checks whether pertinent data, such as history, physical examination and consultation, have been recorded in a problem-oriented fashion. For

PEDIATRICIAN CHART REVIEW FORM

Name of Patient _____ Pediatrician_____

Registration No. _____ Evaluator _____

Date of Birth _____

Date of Last Visit_____

Total No. of Visits Appts. _____ Walk-in _____

NON NEGOTIABLES

For Each Health Maintenance

	Complete		Not Done
Growth Sheet with Entries			
Lab Sheet Urine			
Hct.			
Sickle Prp.			
Vision Screening–Over age 5			
Audiometric Screening–Over age 5			
Immunization Oral Polio #1			
Health Oral Polio #2			
Maintenance Oral Polio #3			
Sheet D.P.T. #1			
D.P.T. #2			
D.P.T. #3			
Rubella Considered			
Measles			
Tine Test			

Pediatrician Chart Review Form (Cont'd.)

HISTORY AND MANAGEMENT

SUBJECTIVE:

	Complete	Incomplete	Not Done
Initial History			
Birth History			
Milestones			
Past Medical History			
Family History			
Subjective Complaints			
OBJECTIVE: Physical Exam			
ASSESSMENT: Well			
Sick			
Routine			
Plan: Immunization			
Treatment			
Consultation			
Referral			
Follow-Up			
Problem Sheet with Entries			
Problem-Oriented Notes			

Check if the following is included at each specified visit

	Always	Sometimes	Never
Temperature			
Blood Pressure (annually over 5)			
Head Circumference (H.M. visit under 1st yr.)			

Check The Following

	Yes	No
Progress Notes Legible	( )	( )
Progress Notes Concise	( )	( )

SUBJECTIVE ASSESSMENT

General Evaluation _____

_____

_____

_____

General Consideration of Care

Excellent _____

Good   _____

Fair   _____

Poor   _____

example, an initial visit would have to include the items listed (birth, history, milestones, family history, etc.).

Subjective Assessment

The reviewer subjectively judges the quality of care given by the practitioners. The protocols are used as a guide.

Method of Review

The Chief of Pediatrics reviews approximately ten charts of the individual practitioners weekly. Reports are sent back to the practitioner for his review. Problem areas are then discussed with each practitioner.

Conclusions

Protocol development and chart evaluation have raised the levels of consciousness on the part of each practitioner. These are particularly valuable when new pediatricians begin to work at the Center. Protocols have provided the pediatrician with standards of care which must be met. The chart evaluation has proven to be an effective means of reviewing the performance of physicians in patient care. Many problems have been detected that otherwise would have continued without this audit. Patient care has definitely improved with the use of the evaluation, protocols and problem-oriented record.

INTERNIST ASSESSMENT
Donald A. Smith, M.D.

Since July 1971 the Medical Care Evaluation Committee has been reviewing one family chart per week, chosen at random. Feedback to the teams has resulted in some improvement of team function. In addition, the process of chart review has accustomed practitioners to the concept of evaluation so that their initial apprehension has diminished greatly.

Despite the advantages of this form of evaluation, two limitations soon became evident. First, only 52 family charts per year could be reviewed (one chart per week). Second, the number of reviewers was limited to a small group, mostly chiefs of the individual services. The majority of the physicians had charts reviewed, but they never had the opportunity to learn from reviewing the charts of others.

To increase the number of charts being audited and the number of physicians involved in medical care assessment, it was decided that each team would audit the family chart of another team once a month. These audits would involve all members of a team. Results of the audits would be given to the audited team and to the Medical Care Evaluation Committee for final review.

In order to assist teams in their audits, the internists have been developing protocols on common diseases to serve as guidelines. These protocols define 1) the data base required for patients with the disease, 2) the minimum note required on each encounter concerning the disease, and 3) the broad goals of therapy. Protocols for such common problems as health maintenance, diabetes, hypertension, gonorrhea and syphilis, urinary tract infection and isoniazid prophylaxis are currently being developed.

The Internist Chart Review Form (see Instructions page 204 and Form page 205) has also been developed to assist internists in their chart audits. This form was necessary in order to be able to compare audits from many different reviewers and to assure that audits by different reviewers would be at equivalent depths of analysis. It has been tested, and is currently undergoing its first use by many reviewing internists. Changes in the format will be made as necessary.

The development of protocols and forms for chart audit by many different reviewers has been exciting and educational. We are eagerly awaiting the results that initiating this new review system will bring.

INSTRUCTIONS FOR USING THE INTERNIST CHART REVIEW FORM

The Internist Chart Review Form is divided into three sections: health maintenance, disease management and overall assessment.

Health maintenance

The health maintenance section is basically a tally sheet to indicate whether specific requirements of health maintenance protocols have been followed. It can be used by a clerical worker indicating by checking the "Y" (yes) box and placing in the box the most recent date when the test or procedure was performed.

> PH   Past history
> FH   Family history
> ROS Review of systems
> PE   Physical exam

Disease Management

This part of the form can only be completed by a physician. The reviewer places in the boxes labeled "Health Problems" those problems which are written on the problem list of the chart. For each of these problems he can then indicate by checking the "Y" (Yes) or "N" (No) column whether the problem is on the problem list and whether there is an adequate data base, assessment, follow-up, and treatment. If any of these areas is inadequate, the reviewer must check "N" and document his opinion by commenting in the adjacent free space. Extra space for further comment can be found in the miscellaneous box at the bottom of the form. In reviewing a chart a physician may find that several problems have not been placed on the problem list. In this case he should write the problem in the health problem box and then check "N" underneath it indicating that the problem was not listed on the problem list in the chart.

Overall Assessment

The physician uses this space for his subjective overall assessment. It is here that the recommendations to the reviewed physician for improvement are made. Equally important comments of praise for good care can be made here as well.

INTERNIST CHART REVIEW

Patient _____   Internist _____
Patient # _____   Date of Review _____
Age _____ Sex _____   Reviewers_____

HEALTH MAINTENANCE

	Adequately done		Comments	TESTS COMPLETED	YES Date	NO
	Yes	No				
PH	(Date)			CHEST X-RAY		
				CBC		
FH				URINALYSIS		
Habits				VDRL		
				SMA 12		
ROS				TINE		
PE				PAP Smear		
				EKG		

DISEASE MANAGEMENT

HEALTH PROBLEMS							
ON PROBLEM LIST	Y N	Y N	Y N	Y N	Y N	Y N	Y N
Adequate Data Bse	Y N	Y N	Y N	Y N	Y N	Y N	Y N
Adequate Assessment	Y N	Y N	Y N	Y N	Y N	Y N	Y N
Adequate F/U treatment	Y N	Y N	Y N	Y N	Y N	Y N	Y N
Miscellaneous							

OVERALL ASSESSMENT

The administrative support systems in operation at MLK as of the spring of 1977 reflect the fact that the center is under the fiscal direction of Montefiore Medical Center. MLK maintains its own computer facilities and has instituted electronic data processing systems to support both the health and administrative services, as described below. Because Montefiore has assumed responsibility for several of the administrative support services, however, MLK's input in some areas has been essentially clerical.

In January 1978, when MLK becomes financially as well as organizationally independent of Montefiore, these systems will have to be developed internally. Some services may be contracted out, subject to HEW approval. What follows is a description of those systems that MLK provides for itself, and brief outlines of those services for which MLK will have to develop systems or alternative means of provision when Montefiore ceases to be its federal grantee in 1978.

ACCOUNTING

The accounting department is primarily responsible for patient service billings and other accounts-receivable management. It also processes the checks covering the accounts-payable (nonsalary expenditures) before forwarding them to Montefiore's department for final processing and payment.

The billing system has been fully automated since 1973. Four kinds of bills are generated by the computer directly from the patient encounter data: one each for Medicare, Medicaid, the 1199 union plan, and self-pay.

If a bill is rejected for reimbursement, for example, from Medicaid, it is automatically resubmitted with clerical corrections if these were indicated or as a self-pay if the patient was not eligible for coverage. In 1976 the initial rejection rate for Medicaid bills (percent returned to the center without payment) was 8 percent, down from 18 percent in 1972–73. It is estimated that with the resubmission procedure the final rejection rate is about 4 percent. The improvement in MLK's rejections occurred primarily from improvements in registration and clerical errors. Medicaid accounted for 92 percent of the center's patient revenues in 1976.

Self-pay are billed on a sliding scale fee-for-service basis, while Medicaid reimburses at flat rates of $50 per center visit. A complete record is maintained for each service provided for every patient encounter, however, so that a detailed fee-for-service charge can be generated for all patients regardless of payment mechanism.

By Kathleen Dalton.

1199 union members are privately charged for 50 percent of the difference between MLK's charge per service provided and the amount covered by their union plan. The amount paid out-of-pocket under this system by union members averages about $2 per clinic visit.

Monthly summaries of the status of all accounts-receivable are prepared for the department with current and year-to-date figures on patient service income. The department aims for a "turnaround time," or lapse between billing and receiving cash, of from six weeks to four months on Medicaid bills. MLK currently records income on a cash basis, that is, revenues are not recognized in the accounts until they are actually received as cash payments. It is anticipated, however, that the more standard accrual basis will be adopted in 1978, whereby revenues will be recognized when the patient is billed, with an allowance also entered to anticipate a set proportion of rejections and/or bad debt.

MIS-cost control is also a function of the accounting department, but it is monitored through departmental summary reports generated by Montefiore reporting system. Monthly and year-to-date figures on actual expenses versus budgeted expenses are recorded by department or unit and by type of expense. The purpose is to identify where and why variances occur from the proposed level of spending. Montefiore also provides periodic income and expense accounts and is reponsible for all external financial reporting. MLK will have to develop capabilities for these services in the near future.

PERSONNEL AND PAYROLL

Personnel is responsible for putting staff on payroll, for maintaining employee files, for processing health service and other employee benefits, and for recruitment.

Employee files include information on status changes, hours worked, accumulated leave, benefits, salary history, vacations, curriculum vitae, licenses, and references. They are maintained manually.

Two sets of time sheets are maintained, one for MLK records and one for Montefiore, which processes the payroll. Employees sign in and out on time sheets kept by department, which are then processed by the payroll persons for the permanent employee files and for the final payroll to be sent to Montefiore.

Recruitment procedures have not changed significantly for the past five years. The policy at MLK (which is also written into the HEW grant specifications) is that new positions be advertised within the agency for approximately one week and then on local community bulletin boards for at least two weeks, in order to provide community people with the first opportunity to fill the position. After a minimum of three weeks the job may be advertised through a newspaper or citiwide agency, but for nonprofessional positions this is rarely necessary.

The payroll function is an example of one of the services currently being provided by Montefiore Hospital that may be temporarily or indefinitely contracted out to a third party, such as a commercial bank.

PURCHASING AND SUPPLIES

The purchasing function is carried out almost entirely by Montefiore staff. A clerical person from MLK is assigned ro receive and record purchase requisitions from MLK's comptroller and pass them on to a Montefiore buyer, who does all of the negotiations for price and delivery.

A perpetual inventory system is used for all MLK supplies, but is currently not maintained by department. Consequently there is no accountability within units or departments for inventory control. MLK is currently working on a departmentally based inventory control system and anticipates its implementation by January 1978.

APPOINTMENTS

Centralized appointment logs are maintained on the computer. Units are provided with a regularly updated printout of the appointment schedules of each of their clinicians. There is no automated capability to coordinate appointments to different clinicians to minimize total visits to the center, but a conscious attempt is made to do this manually with Medicare patients because of the difficulties that they experience in getting to the clinic.

The card for the appointment record contains basic information, such as name, registration number, insurance coverage, and doctor. Diagnosis and treatment are entered after the visit and the same card becomes the encounter record for that visit.

Each day a list of appointments for two days hence is printed out and sent to each department. Another is sent to medical records so that all necessary records are pulled and forwarded to the department by the beginning of the following day. Persons with long-range appointments (more than 12 weeks in advance) are sent reminders shortly before the appointment date.

No-shows are recorded on the appointment record and entered into the patient's permanent file. Family health workers are responsible for follow-up on all broken appointments and no-shows.

Transportation services are provided by the center for those who are coordinated with the appointment system.

The appointment system is estimated to be 90 percent accurate. The batch-processing mode used by the MLK's computer facilities prevents the use of totally current records when appointments are made, thereby resulting in some accidental double-booking. If an on-line computer system were used (with terminals) each time a free slot was searched for in a clinician's schedule, the schedule would be current and updated. By relying on periodic appointment printouts, some double-booking is unavoidable.

REGISTRATION

The registration system is fully computerized. An eligible new patient is given a permanent registration number and card for him- or herself and one for each family member at the initial visit. Although all family members are registered at that time, the computer has a flagging mechanism to indicate which persons have actually been seen at the center in order to distinguish between active and inactive registrants.

Health and social questionnaires are administered at the time of registration and data are included on the permanent patient record. Payment status and financial statements are updated at least every six months.

Patient's rights information and other brochures about the center are distributed in English and Spanish, at the time of registration.

All persons living within the center's catchment area are eligible to register for the center's services. Because of financial difficulties encountered from the low collection rate for self-pay and some third-party-insured individuals, however, an unofficial procedure has developed whereby only Medicaid, Medicare, or fully covered third-party insured persons are registered for comprehensive, family-oriented team services. Other individuals are registered separately and treated for episodic emergency care and limited physician services only.

The practice of maintaining what are effectively two registered populations for two kinds of care has evolved informally over time. It is an ad hoc response to increasing pressures on the organization to support its operations through the patient revenues that it generates. Whether or not this practice will continue depends upon basic fiscal and managerial policy issues that will be addressed as the governance of MLK is transferred to the community board.

ELECTRONIC DATA PROCESSING (EDP)

MLK's data processing unit currently utilizes an IBM system 360-30, on third-party lease. The registration, appointment, patient information, and billing systems described previously occupy approximately 40 percent of its available processing time.

In addition to these services, EDP provides an extensive lab reporting system, maintaining reports on tests done in-house, and an automatic notification procedure to indicate if results are pending from tests sent out to other facilities.

A Management Information System (MIS) generates monthly utilization reports by team and by clinician, designed primarily for quantitative evaluation of clinical services. It also generates quarterly management reports and utilization statistics required by HEW. Patient encounter data are presented on an activity per team/per clinician/per session/ or per time period basis; present facilities do not have the capability to analyze by diagnosis or by treatment.

Approximately 10 percent of the EDP department's time is spent in program development. An attempt to implement patient information systems, organized chronologically, of a patient's history, tests, diagnoses, and so on, is currently underway. This will alleviate problems of discontinuity created by MLK's participation in the Montefiore residency program, with its consequent high physician turnover.

MLK also provides limited data processing services to members of the New York Association of Neighborhood Health Centers.

BIBLIOGRAPHY

Aiken, Michael. 1970. "The Distribution of Community Power: Structural Bases and Social Consequences." In *The Structure of Community Power*, ed. Michael Aiken and Paul Mott, pp. 487–525. New York: Random House.

———, R. Dewar, N. DiTomasi, J. Hage, and G. Zeitz. 1975. *Coordinating Human Services*. San Francisco: Jossey Bass.

Argyris, Chris. 1964. *Integrating the Individual and the Organization*. New York: Wiley.

———. 1970. *Intervention Theory and Method: A Behavioral Science View*. Reading, Mass.: Addison-Wesley.

———. 1971. "Management Information Systems: The Challenge to Rationality." *Management Science* 17: 275–92.

Beckhard, Richard. 1969. *Organizational Development: Strategies and Models*. Reading, Mass.: Addison-Wesley.

———. 1972. "Organizational Issues in the Team Delivery of Comprehensive Health Care." *Milbank Memorial Fund Quarterly* (July 1): pp. 287–316.

———. 1974. "ABS in Health Care Systems: Who Needs It?" *Journal of Applied Behavioral Science* 10:1, 93–106.

———. 1975. "Organization Development in Large Systems." In *The Laboratory Method of Changing and Learning*, ed. K. Benne, L. Bradford, J. Gibb, R. Lippitt. Palo Alto, Calif.: Science and Behavior Books.

———, Harold Wise, Irwin Rubin, and Aileen L. Kyte. 1974. *Making Health Teams Work*. Cambridge, Mass.: Ballinger.

Blau, Peter. 1955. *Dynamics of Bureaucracy*. Chicago: University of Chicago Press.

———. 1956. *Bureaucracy in Modern Society*. New York: Random House.

Braybrooke, D., and C. E. Lindblom. 1963. *A Strategy of Decision*. New York: Free Press.

Burns, Thomas, and G. M. Stalker. 1961. *The Management of Innovation*. London: Fairstock.

Carlson, Rick. 1975. *The End of Medicine*. New York: Wiley.

Chandler, Alfred. 1962. *Strategy and Structure*. Cambridge, Mass.: MIT Press.

Chapple, Eliot, and Leonard Sayles. 1961. *The Measure of Management*. New York: Macmillan.

Cherkasky, Martin. 1949. "Hospital Home Care Program." *American Journal of Public Health* 39 (February): 29–30.

———. 1971. "Doctors and Community Control." In *Doctors and Community Control, Transaction and Studies of the College of Physicians in Philadelphia* 38: 212–20.

Dalton, Melville. 1959. *Men Who Manage: Fusions of Feeling and Theory in Administration.* New York. Wiley.

Davis, Stanley. 1976. "Trends in the Organization of Multinational Corporations." *Columbia Journal of World Business* (summer): 59.

Delbecq, Andre. 1967. "The Management of Decision Making Within the Firm: Three Strategies for Three Types of Decision Making." *Academy of Management Journal* (December): 329–39.

Deutsch, Martin. 1973. *The Resolution of Conflict.* New Haven: Yale University Press.

Drucker, Peter. 1973. *Management.* New York: Harper & Row.

Emery, Fred, and Eric Trist. 1965. "The Causal Texture of Organizational Environments." *Human Relations* 18:21–32.

Etzioni, Amitai. 1961. *Comparative Analysis of Complex Organizations.* New York: Free Press.

———. 1969. *The Semi-Professions and Their Organization.* New York: Free Press.

———. 1975. "Accountability in Health Administration." In *Education for Health Administration*, vol. 2. Ann Arbor, Mich.: Health Administration Press.

Evan, W. M., 1966. "The Organization-Set: Toward a Theory of Interorganizational Relations." In *Approaches to Organization Design*, ed. J. D. Thompson. Pittsburgh: University of Pittsburgh Press.

Feinhold, E. 1971. "A Political Scientist's View of the Neighborhood Health Center as a Social Institution." *Medical Care* 8:108–15.

Friedson, E. 1970. "Professional Dominance: The Social Structure of Medical Care." New York: Atherton Press.

Fry, Ronald, Bernard Lech, and Irwin Rubin. 1974. "Working with the Primary Care Team: The First Intervention." In *Making Health Teams Work*, ed. H. Wise, R. Beckhard, I. Rubin, and A. Kyte. Cambridge, Mass.: Ballinger.

Galbraith, Jay. 1973. *Designing Complex Organizations.* Reading, Mass.: Addison-Wesley.

Geiger, H. J. 1974. "Community Control or Community Conflict?" In *Neighborhood Health Centers*, ed. R. M. Hollister, B. Kramer, and S. Bellin. Lexington, Mass.: Lexington Books.

Georgopoulos, Basil S. 1975. *Hospital Organization Research: Review and Source Book*. Philadelphia: Saunders.

————, and F. C. Mann. 1962. *The Community General Hospital*. New York: Macmillan.

Gerstner, Louis. 1972. "Can Strategic Planning Pay Off?" *Business Horizons*, December, pp. 5-16.

Gordon, J. B. 1969. "The Politics of Community Medicine Projects: A Conflict Analysis." *Medical Care* 4:419-28.

Gouldner, Alvin. 1954. *Patterns of Industrial Bureaucracy*. New York: Free Press.

Greiner, Larry. 1972. "Evolution and Revolution as Organizations Grow." *Harvard Business Review* (July-August).

Hackman, Richard. 1976. "Group Influences on Individuals in Organizations." In *Handbook of Industrial and Organizational Psychology*, ed. M. D. Dunnette. Chicago: Rand McNally.

Hage, J., and Michael Aiken. 1967. "Program Change and Organization Properties: A Comparative Analysis." *American Journal of Sociology* (March).

————. 1970. *Social Change in Complex Organizations*. New York: Random House.

Hedberg, B., P. Nystrom, and W. Starbuck. 1976. "Camping on Seesaws: Prescriptions for a Self-designing Organization." *Administrative Science Quarterly* 21, no. 1 (March): 41-65.

Helfgot, J. 1974. "Professional Reform Organizations and the Symbolic Representation of the Poor." *American Social Review* 37: 431-95.

Hollister, Robert M., B. M. Kramer, and S. S. Bellin, eds. 1974. *Neighborhood Health Centers*. Lexington, Mass.: Lexington Books.

Hornstein, Harvey, B. Benedict, W. Burke, M. Hornstein, and R. Lewicki. 1971. *Social Intervention: A Behavioral Science Approach*. New York: Macmillan.

Hornstein, Harvey, and Noel Tichy. 1976. "Developing Organization Development for Multinational Corporations." *Columbia Journal of World Business* (summer).

Hrebiniak, Lawrence. 1977. *Complex Organizations*. St. Paul, Minn.: West.

Hutchinson, John. 1976. "Evolving Organizational Forms." *Columbia Journal of World Business* (summer): 48.

Illich, Ivan. 1974. *Medical Nemesis*. London: Calder and Boyars.

Katz, Daniel, and Robert Kahn. 1966. *Social Psychology of Organizations*. New York: Wiley.

Kelley, H., and J. Thibaut. 1968. "Group Problem Solving." In *Handbook of Social Psychology*, ed. G. Lindzey and E. Aronson. Reading, Mass.: Addison-Wesley.

Kissick, William. 1970. "Health Policy Directions for the 1970's." *New England Journal of Medicine* 282, no. 24 (July): 1343–54.

————, and Samuel Miller. 1976. "Organization of Personal Health Services." In *Resource Book on Health and Behavioral Sciences in Health Administration*, ed. Kent Peterson. Washington, D.C.: Association of University Programs in Health Administration.

Kubicek, Thomas. 1972. "Organization Planning: What It Is and How to Do It. Part I. The Organizational Audit." *Cost and Management* (January).

Lawler, Edward. 1971. *Pay and Organizational Performance: A Psychological View.* New York: McGraw-Hill.

————. 1976. "Control Systems in Organizations." In *Handbook of Industrial and Organizational Psychology*, ed. Marvin Dunnette. Chicago: Rand McNally.

Lawrence, Paul, and Jay Lorsch. 1962. *Organization and Environment: Managing Integration.* Homewood, Ill.: Richard D. Irwin.

————. 1967. *Organization and Environment.* Cambridge, Mass.: Harvard University Press.

————. 1969. *Developing Organizations.* Reading, Mass.: Addison-Wesley.

Levine, S., and P. White. 1961. "Exchange and Interorganizational Relationships." *Administrative Science Quarterly* J, no. 4.

Lewin, Kurt. 1948. *Resolving Social Conflicts.* New York: Harper and Brothers.

————. 1965. "Group Decision and Social Change." In *Handbook of Organizations*, ed. James March, pp. 1144–70. Chicago: Rand McNally.

Lipset, S. M., M. A. Trow, and J. S. Coleman. 1956. *Union Democracy.* Glencoe, Ill.: Free Press.

Lloyd, William B., and Harold B. Wise. 1968. "The Montefiore Experience." *Bulletin of the New York Academy of Medicine,* 2d ser. 44 (November):1353–62.

MacCrimmon, Kenneth, and Donald Taylor. 1976. "Decision-making and Problem Solving." In *Handbook of Industrial and Organizational Psychology*, ed. Marvin Dunnette. Chicago: Rand McNally.

March, James, and Herbert Simon. 1958. *Organizations.* New York: Wiley.

————. 1962. *Organizations.* New York: Macmillan.

Dr. Martin Luther King, Jr. Health Center. 1970. *Dr. Martin Luther King, Jr. Health Center Fourth Annual Report.*

Mechanic, David. 1969. "Future of General Medical Practice in the U.S." *Inquiry* 6, no. 2, 17–26.

————. 1972. "Social Psychological Factors Affecting the Presentation of Bodily Complaints." *New England Journal of Medicine* 286 (May): 1132–39.

Mintzberg, Henry. 1976a. "Patterns in Strategy Formation" (working paper). McGill University.

————. 1976b. "The Structure of Unstructural Decision Processes." *Administrative Science Quarterly* 21, no. 2.

Morehead, Mildred, and R. Donaldson. 1970. "Comparisons Between OEO Neighborhood Health Centers and Other Health Care Providers of Rating of the Quality of Care." Paper presented before the Medical Care Section, Annual Meeting of the American Public Health Association, Houston, Tex., October 25–29.

Morehead, Mildred, Rose Donaldson, and Mary Seravalli. 1971. "Comparisons Between OEO Neighborhood Health Centers and Other Health Care Providers of Ratings of the Quality of Health Care." *American Journal of Public Health* 61, 7 (July).

Moynihan, Daniel P. 1969. *Maximum Feasible Misunderstanding: Community Action in the War on Poverty.* New York: Free Press.

Newman, W. A., and J. P. Logan. 1955. *Management of Expanding Enterprises.* New York: Columbia University Press.

Newman, H. William. 1967. "Shaping the Master Strategy of Your Firm." *California Management Review* (spring): 86.

Newman, William. 1971–72. "Strategy and Management Structure." *Journal of Business Policy* (winter): 56–66.

Parker, Alberta. 1972. "The Team Approach to Primary Health Care." Neighborhood Health Center Monograph Series no. 3. University Extension, University of California, Berkeley.

Pearse, I. H., and L. H. Crocker. 1943. *The Peckham Experiment: A Study in the Living Structure of Society.* London: Allen & Unwin.

Perrow, C. 1965. "Hospital Technology, Structures and Goals." In *Handbook of Organizations*, ed. J. G. March. Chicago: Rand McNally.

————. 1970. *Organizational Analysis: A Sociological View.* Belmont, Calif.: Wadsworth.

————. 1972. *Complex Organizations.* Glenview, Ill.: Scott, Foresman.

Reed, Jeanne M. 1974a. "The Problem Oriented Record." In *Dr. Martin Luther King, Jr. Health Center Annual Report, 1974*, ed. Wendy Singley, pp. 181–87.

———. 1974b. "Quality of Care." In *Dr. Martin Luther King, Jr. Health Center Annual Report, 1974*, ed. Wendy Singley.

Rubin, Irwin, M. S. Plovnick, and R. Fry. 1975. *Improving the Coordination of Care: A Program for Health Team Development*. Cambridge, Mass.: Ballinger.

Rubin, Lilian. 1967. "Maximum Feasible Participation: The Origins, Implications, and Present Status." *Poverty and Human Resources Abstracts*, 2: 5–18.

Sayles, Leonard R. 1958. *Behavior of Industrial Work Groups*. New York: Wiley.

Schein, Edgar. 1968. "Organizational Socialization and the Profession of Management." *Industrial Management Review* 9: 1–16.

———. 1970. *Organizational Psychology*, 2d ed. Englewood Cliffs, N.J.: Prentice-Hall.

———. 1971. "The Individual, the Organization, and the Career: A Conceptual Scheme." *Journal of Applied Behavioral Science*, pp. 401–26.

Schorr, Elizabeth, and Joseph English. 1968. "Background Context and Significant Issues in Neighborhood Health Center Programs." *Milbank Memorial Fund Quarterly* 66, no. 3, part 1 (July).

Scott, W. Richard. 1965. "Field Methods in the Study of Organizations." In *Handbook of Organizations*, ed. James March. Chicago: Rand McNally.

Selznick, P. 1949. *TVA and the Grass Roots*. Berkeley: University of California Press.

Shortell, Steven M. 1977. "The Role of Environment in a Configuration Theory of Organization." *Human Relations* 30: 275–302.

Siegel, Benjamin. 1974. "Organization of the Primary Care Team." *Pediatric Clinics of North America* 21, no. 2 (May).

Silver, George A. 1958. "Beyond General Practice: The Health Team." *Yale Journal of Biology and Medicine* 31, no. 1 (September).

———. 1963. *Family Medical Care: A Design for Health Maintenance*. Cambridge, Mass.: Ballinger.

———. 1969. "What Has Been Learned from the Neighborhood Health Centers." Excerpts from "What Has Been Learned About the Delivery of Health Care Services to the Ghetto?" *Medicine in the Ghetto*. New York: Appleton-Century-Crofts, pp. 65–72.

Simon, Herbert. 1967. "The Business School: A Problem in Organizational Design." *Journal of Management Studies* 4: 1–16.

Singley, Wendy, ed. 1973. Dr. Martin Luther King, Jr. Health Center, *Sixth Annual Report*.

Smith, Deloris. 1973. "Interview with Deloris Smith." In *Dr. Martin Luther King, Jr. Health Center, Sixth Annual Report*, ed. Wendy Singley.

———, and Edward Martin. 1973. "Evaluation of Quality of Case Delivery by Ambulatory Health Care Teams." Unpublished.

Smith, Donald. 1974. "Internist Assessment." In *Dr. Martin Luther King, Jr. Health Center, Sixth Report*.

Sparer, Gerald, and A. Anderson. 1972. "Cost of Services at Neighborhood Health Centers: A Comparative Analysis." *New England Journal of Medicine* 286 (June 8), 1241–45.

Tichy, Noel. 1973. "An Analysis of Clique Formation and Structure in Organizations." *Administrative Science Quarterly* 18, no. 2, 194–208.

———. 1976. "Community Control of Health Services." *Health Education Monographs* 4, no. 2 (summer).

———. 1978. "Organizational Networks, Coalitions and Cliques." In *Handbook of Organization Design*, ed. W. Starbuck. Elsevier Press.

———, and Richard Beckhard. 1976. "Applied Behavioral Science for Health Administrators." Working Paper 879–76. Sloan School of Management, Massachusetts Institute of Technology.

Thompson, J. D. 1967. *Organizations in Action*. New York: McGraw-Hill.

Thompson, James, and William McEwen. 1958. "Organizational Goals and Environment: Goal Setting as an Interaction Process." *American Sociological Review* 23, no. 1: 23–30.

Torrens, Paul. 1971. "Administrative Problems of Neighborhood Health Centers." *Medical Care* 9: 487–97.

Tushman, Michael, and David Nadler. 1976. "Basic Concepts of and Approaches to Organizational Structure." Working paper, Graduate School of Business, Columbia University.

Vroom, V. H., and D. W. Yetton. 1973. *Leadership and Decision-Making*. Pittsburgh: University of Pittsburgh Press.

Walton, Richard. 1969. *Interpersonal Piecemaking: Confrontation and Third Party Consultations*. Reading, Mass.: Addison-Wesley.

Weber, Max. 1946. *From Max Weber: Essays in Sociology*, ed. H. K. Gerth and C. W. Mills. New York: Oxford University Press.

———. 1964. *The Theory of Social and Economic Organization*. Translated by Henderson and Parsons. New York: Free Press.

Weick, Karl. 1969. *Social Psychology of Organizing*. Reading, Mass.: Addison-Wesley.

White, Kerr. 1973. "Life and Death and Medicine." *Scientific American*, September 1973.

Wise, Harold. 1966. "Proposal for Demonstration and Training Research Grant." USOE Community Action Program, Montefiore Hospital as Sponsor. Original MLK proposal.

————. 1968. "Montefiore Hospital Neighborhood Medical Care Demonstration." *Milbank Memorial Fund Quarterly* 66, Pt. I, 287–307.

————. 1970, 1971. Dr. Martin Luther King, Jr. Health Center, *Fourth and Fifth Annual Reports.*

————. 1972. "The Primary Care Health Team." *Archives of Internal Medicine* 130 (September): 438–44.

————, L. S. Levin, and R. T. Kurahawa. "Community Development and Health Education: Community Organization as a Health Tactic." *Milbank Memorial Fund Quarterly* 46: 325.

Wise, Harold, Richard Beckhard, Irwin Rubin, and Aileen L. Kyte. 1974. *Making Health Teams Work.* Cambridge, Mass.: Ballinger.

Wrapp, Edward. 1967. "Good Managers Don't Make Policy Decisions." *Harvard Business Review* 45, no. 5, pp. 91–99.

Zelditch, M. 1969. "Some Methodological Problems of Field Studies." In *Issues in Participant Observation: A Text and Reader*, ed. G. T. McCall and J. L. Simmons. Reading, Mass.: Addison-Wesley.

SUBJECT INDEX

NOEL M. TICHY is associate professor in the management of organizations area of the Graduate School of Business, Columbia University, and senior research associate at the Center for Policy Research, Inc.

Dr. Tichy has published widely in the area of organizational behavior and the applied behavioral sciences. His articles have appeared in the *Administrative Science Quarterly*, *Human Relations*, *Group and Organizational Studies*, *Journal of Applied Behavioral Sciences*, *Columbia Journal of World Business*, and the *Academy of Management Review*.

Dr. Tichy holds a B.A. from Colgate University and a Ph.D. from Columbia University. He is a member of the American Psychological Association, the Academy of Management, the NTL-Institute of Applied Behavioral Sciences, and Sigma Xi, the Scientific Research Society of America.

ACCOUNTABILITY IN HEALTH FACILITIES

Harry I. Greenfield

BEHAVIORAL SCIENCE TECHNIQUES: An Annotated
Bibliography for Health Professionals

Monique K. Tichy

COMMUNITY CONTROL OF ECONOMIC DEVELOPMENT:
The Boards of Directors of Community Development
Corporations

Rita Mae Kelly

THE DESIGN OF A HEALTH MAINTENANCE ORGANIZATION:
A Handbook for Practitioners

Allan Easton

HEALTH CARE GUIDANCE: Commercial Health Insurance
and National Health Policy

Carol Klaperman Morrow

THE ORGANIZATION AND OPERATION OF NEIGHBORHOOD
COUNCILS: A Practical Guide

Howard H. Hallman